Fred DeVito and Elisabeth Halfpapp

BARRE
FITNESS

Fred DeVito and Elisabeth Halfpapp

part of the founding team of exhale; co-creators of Core Fusion® Fitness Program

BARRE FITNESS

Barre Exercises You Can Do Anywhere
for Flexibility, Core Strength, and a Lean Body

FAIR WINDS

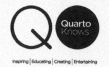

Brimming with creative inspiration, how-to projects, and useful information to enrich your everyday life, Quarto Knows is a favorite destination for those pursuing their interests and passions. Visit our site and dig deeper with our books into your area of interest: Quarto Creates, Quarto Cooks, Quarto Homes, Quarto Lives, Quarto Drives, Quarto Explores, Quarto Gifts, or Quarto Kids.

First Published in 2016 by Fair Winds Press, an imprint of The Quarto Group,
100 Cummings Center, Suite 265-D, Beverly, MA 01915, USA.
T (978) 282-9590 F (978) 283-2742 QuartoKnows.com

Fair Winds Press titles are also available at discount for retail, wholesale, promotional, and bulk purchase. For details, contact the Special Sales Manager by email at specialsales@quarto.com or by mail at The Quarto Group, Attn: Special Sales Manager, 100 Cummings Center, Suite 265-D, Beverly, MA 01915, USA.

ISBN: 978-1-59233-691-3

Digital edition published in 2016
eISBN: 978-1-62788-787-8

Library of Congress Cataloging-in-Publication Data

DeVito, Fred.
  Barre fitness : barre exercises you can do anywhere for flexibility, core strength, and a lean body / Fred Devito and Elisabeth Halfpapp, part of the founding team of Exhale and co-creators of Core Fusion Fitness Program.
    pages cm
  Includes index.
  ISBN 978-1-59233-691-3 -- ISBN 978-1-62788-787-8 (eISBN)
  1. Exercise. 2. Ballet. I. Title.
  GV481.D48 2015
  613.7--dc23
                              2015025995

Design: Lori Wendin
Page Layout: Laura H. Couallier, Laura Herrmann Design
Photography: Luciana Pampalone
Photographed on location at The Exhale Studio, The Manhattan House, New York City

"If it doesn't challenge you, it doesn't change you" is a trademark of Fred Devito.

The information in this book is for educational purposes only. It is not intended to replace the advice of a physician or medical practitioner. Please see your health care provider before beginning any new health program.

To our parents, who have been instrumental in supporting our career paths:

Christa Halfpapp, Ben Halfpapp, Fred L. DeVito, Nancy DeVito

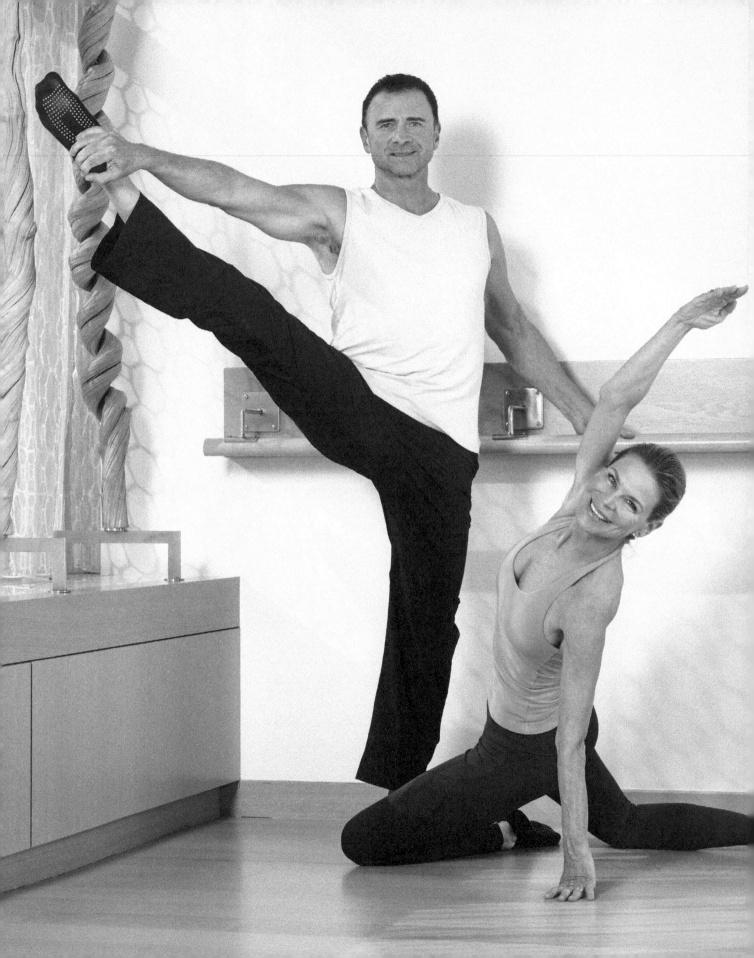

CONTENTS

___

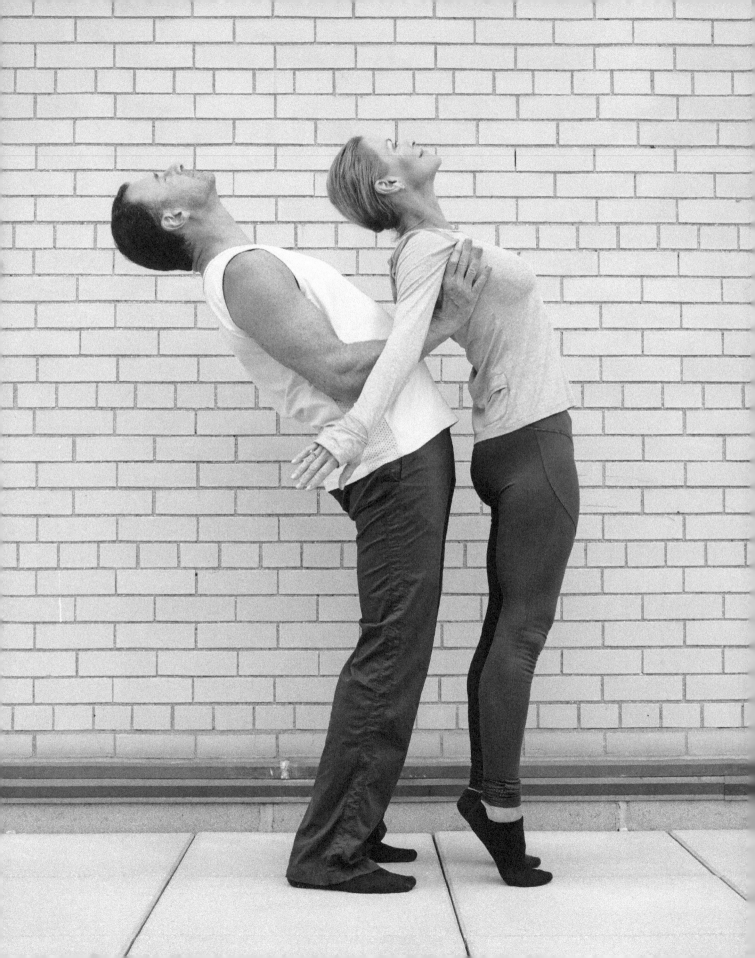

INTRODUCTION

Welcome to our world of barre fitness! We are excited to have this opportunity to share our life's work with you in the pages of this book. Your background with fitness may fall anywhere on the spectrum, from couch potato or weekend warrior to serious dancer or athlete. Whatever the case may be, these exercises may be the missing link in your effort to improve your fitness level and healthy lifestyle. Expect to be challenged in ways you haven't imagined, because **if it doesn't challenge you, it doesn't change you**. Results occur within weeks of committing to the program outlined in the chapters ahead. Are you ready?

HISTORY OF BARRE FITNESS

This is a book born from the barre class industry, one of the fastest-growing segments in the exercise class market to hit the fitness industry in the past 10 years. Our collective experience of more than 60 years of barre class teaching, teacher training, business development, and program execution began in a brownstone building on the Upper East Side of New York City in a little five-room boutique fitness studio called the Lotte Berk Method, which ultimately became the birthplace of this incredible movement technique.

The genius behind the system, Lotte Berk, was a German modern dancer who injured her back while performing in the 1950s. With the help of her physical therapists and her knowledge of movement through dance, she created and started teaching an exercise technique called Rehabilitative Exercise on Manchester Street in London. Our mentor and teacher, Lydia Bach, studied with Lotte in the late 1960s before she came to NYC and honored the creator by opening a studio, in the early 1970s, named The Lotte Berk Method. Her studio was only for women, and after a "Best-of Award" in *New York Magazine,* she was flooded with calls from people wanting to take her barre classes.

The Lotte Berk Method was not gaining popularity because it was a new fitness fad—it was therapeutic as well, especially for the back and abdominals. Lydia worked with the doctors of the rehabilitative departments in what is now Weill Cornell Medical College in New York City and New York University hospitals, detailing how bracing and stabilization of the back and abdominals (a cornerstone of barre class at the Lotte Berk Method studio) was like advanced physical therapy. As a result, they would send their post–physical therapy patients to the Lotte Berk Method studio.

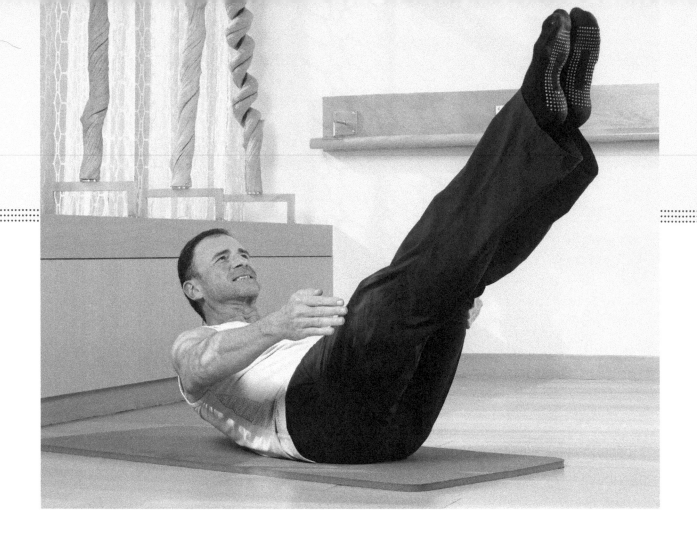

OUR BACKGROUND IN BARRE

Elisabeth (or Lis) began teaching at the Lotte Berk Method studio in 1980 after graduating from the Hartford School of Ballet Teacher Training program (trained in the Vaganova Technique, which is the Kirov Ballet's system) and dancing with the Mercer Ballet, Princeton Ballet (now American Repertory Ballet), and Hartford Ballet. Within a year, she was promoted to the studio manager and began overseeing an incredible thriving business while still teaching and training all the teachers.

While dating Lis, Fred taught public school physical education and adult personal training in health clubs in New York City. After seeing the physical results of barre fitness on their wives

and girlfriends, men became interested in joining barre classes, too. Thus, Fred began teaching at the Lotte Berk Method as the first male ever allowed inside that female inner sanctum.

In the 1970s and early 1980s, the Lotte Berk Method had a strong feminine quality to not only the exercises and positions but also in the language and inferences. For example, the classic term for the butt was "seat" and students were told to pull in their "tummies." Upper body exercises were lacking in the class. There were a few isometric chest pumps along with countless, fatiguing straight arm circles using 1- or 2-pound (455 to 910 g) weights—that was the arm section

The Lotte Berk Method became a hallmark for high achievers in the Upper East Side social set of New York City. It became very chic and exclusive to be a part of a workout program such as barre fitness, and soon class appointments came at a premium.

of the class. Under Lydia's tutelage, we began to subtly evolve and modernize the technique, making the class more gender neutral and therapeutic. Working with people of all body types and people with different types of injuries and limitations gave us practical insight for working the body safely and efficiently.

Now, after spending more than a combined 60 years in this industry, we have seen it develop and grow to be one of the most popular classes both live, online, and in DVD format, with many of our former teachers and students now leading their own barre business in either the franchise or boutique studio models.

In 2002, along with two other colleagues, Annbeth Eschbach and Julia Sutton, we founded exhale, a brand that launched as a mind/body/spa company. With exhale came the birth of our company's proprietary barre class, Core Fusion. In our transition from Lotte Berk Method to exhale and Core Fusion, we had a chance to pause and determine what was important to us both inside and outside the classroom. Our classroom programming focus became mind-body exploration. By incorporating a yogic mentality, we began teaching how to focus on the breath and move from a place of wisdom instead of ego. You will learn to let go of the need to compete or compare when you exercise and make the experience more

inner and personal rather than about the superficial and outside stimuli. Our discovery, after all, was that barre fitness is a moving meditation and a lifestyle practice, not just a class that lifts your butt and firms your thighs and abdominals! So yes—you can have it all!

WHAT IS BARRE FITNESS?

A *barre* is typically a fixed and sturdy horizontal pole attached to a wall that dancers use for balance, stability, and support as they perform specific moves for dance training. But you do not need an actual barre or experience as a dancer to do these exercises.

The barre exercises described in this book will teach and demonstrate the proper form for the most classic barre positions for the legs and gluteals. You will also use the barre to brace yourself during abdominal exercises. Some moves are compound, using double leg action, and some are single leg, which means you would need to complete each side with the same amount of emphasis and focus.

For each of these movements, we provide a position setup and an easy-to-follow progression. As the level of the exercise advances, your priority is to make your position and form more precise and more accurate, before then adding repetitions.

Barre fitness exercises the body in a balanced way, improving strength, core stability, flexibility, and bone density. It also reduces stress and improves your sense of well-being.

The exercise positions are designed to target the major muscles of the body, such as your abdominals, thighs, glutes, chest, shoulders, back, and arm muscles. The strength work and flexibility training are meant to challenge you. Push yourself! We take a balanced approach to the workout that enables you to realize a strong core and a supple, vibrant, and youthful body.

WHAT YOU NEED

If you don't have a barre at home, you can use a sturdy high-back chair or counter top. Some of the exercises, especially for the abdominals, are done on the floor using an exercise mat. Wear comfortable clothes and either wear grip socks or exercise in bare feet to avoid slipping. If you have a mirror, you can use it to check your position in your side view. Don't forget to stay hydrated and take breaks when you need to.

BENEFITS OF BARRE FITNESS

Exercise doesn't have to beat you down to be effective. On the contrary, people who suffer from overuse injuries are better able to heal in a barre class. We use props, belts, blocks, resistance bands, and a light free weight section to allow for steady progress over time. Men and women who come in exhibiting sports injuries feel less pain and more flexibility. Barre fitness becomes therapy for people rehabilitating minor injuries as long as they participate consistently in the program with commitment. In fitness-minded folks from weekend warriors to professional athletes, the barre exercise system produces real results.

Barre fitness exercises the body in a balanced way, improving strength, core stability, flexibility, and bone density. It also reduces stress and improves your sense of well-being.

HOW BARRE WILL TRANSFORM YOUR BODY

When barre exercises are taught with a focus on proper position and alignment and are performed with a focused effort at least three times per week, you can expect to see the following results.

Increase Bone Density

As women age, they will start to see a decrease in their estrogen levels, which can lead to a loss of bone density. This can begin prior to menopause, and within five years after menopause, women lose as much as 25 percent of bone density. This can lead to an increased risk of the development of osteoporosis, a disorder in which bones become fragile and more likely to break. Older adults with osteoporosis are most likely to suffer bone breakage, which severely limits their mobility and independence.

You can take steps to increase your bone strength and reduce your chances of having a fracture. You can combine calcium and vitamin D supplements with weight-bearing and weight-training exercises. Most barre exercises require standing on either one or both legs, using your own body weight as resistance. The more that a muscle pulls on a bone during physical activity, the greater the bone density needs to be for stability. You can adjust the barre exercises in our book in both intensity and duration with a progressive approach to help improve bone density gradually.

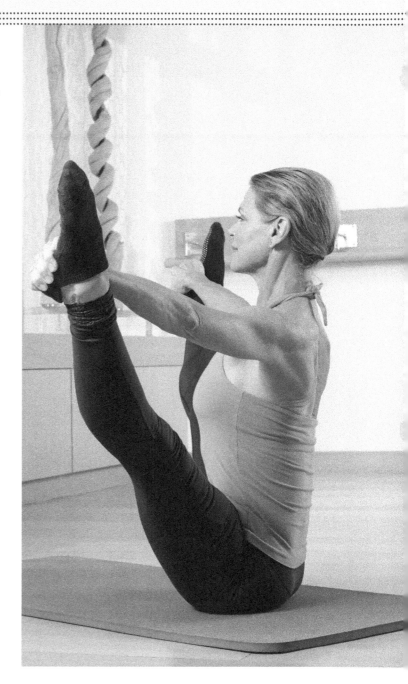

Increase Muscle Density

We lose about 4 percent of our muscle density every year unless we do something to prevent that from happening. Your muscles are the engines of your body, providing work, producing energy, and burning calories. Having muscles that are dense and strong will help you to maintain a higher-than-average resting metabolic rate (RMR) so that you have the potential to burn calories 24/7, even when your body is at rest. This is an important factor if you are trying to lose or maintain your body weight. Weight-bearing exercises that strengthen your muscles will ignite your RMR and turn you into a calorie-burning furnace! Cardio is important, but it is the muscle tissue in your body that burns the calories in any activity, whether it's walking, running, biking, or swimming. Barre exercises use your own body weight as resistance for strengthening exercises, and muscle density improves over time with strength training. Muscles that are dense and lean require more fuel (calories) to do what is asked at a higher level of efficiency.

Improve Muscle Elasticity

Muscular elasticity is maintained and sometimes improved with flexibility training. Muscles will lose elasticity as you age, and as muscles shorten, the tendons that connect the muscle to the bone can be compromised, leading to inflammation (tendonitis). When your muscles have an elastic property to them, this increased suppleness will allow your muscles to stretch without strain, and this keeps your body feeling more youthful. If you are active in any sport, your range of motion is important. Barre fitness promotes flexibility training as much as the strengthening exercises. And you can improve your flexibility over time using the three Ps: **Persistence**, **Perseverance**, and **Patience**.

Body Shaping

You will obtain long lean thighs, a high round butt, and flat abdominals with barre fitness. Strengthening work is complemented by stretches that elongate the muscles, especially the legs. The strengthening exercises for the glutes, for example, involve moving your leg against the resistance of the pelvis braced by your core, thereby working your butt. Many of the movements, from forearm plank to the curl position, involve "pulling in" the abdominal wall to produce flat abdominals. As your core gets stronger, you can increase the difficulty of your exercises, resulting in better and faster results.

With **persistence**, **perseverance**, and **patience**, you will gradually balance out your muscular system, reduce chronic aches and pains, raise your level of fitness, and discover the joy of movement that you had in your youth.

Therapeutic Benefits

When you perform barre exercises with a careful focus on position and alignment, your exercise mirrors a physical therapy session. We are more concerned with the quality of your movements than the quantity of your movements. We would rather you focus on the sections of the book that really challenge you than have you perform only the movements that you like to do and are good at doing. Following the principle that a chain is only as strong as its weakest link, work on the exercises that challenge you, and you will see improvements. With **persistence**, **perseverance**, and **patience**, you will gradually balance out your muscular system, reduce chronic aches and pains, raise your level of fitness, and discover the joy of movement that you had in your youth.

Pregnancy—Before, During, and After

When you become pregnant, you will go through major physical changes. Many exercise programs can be too stressful or intense for a pregnant woman, but barre fitness is one that you can do successfully and effectively as your body develops during pregnancy and recovers post-pregnancy. With your doctor's permission, a pregnant woman can perform these exercises four or five times per week with modifications on intensity and duration. It is important that you focus on minimizing your exertion and exercise with a maintenance plan approach. As your body changes, so will your exercise needs. Women have successfully performed nine months of barre fitness and seen benefits such as reduced discomfort (especially in the lower back), increased energy, regulated mood swings, and faster postpartum recovery. After your delivery, you will have strong arms and upper body to carry and lift your baby, whose weight increases every week.

LET'S GET STARTED

With *Barre Fitness*, you have all the tools you need to complete a rigorous yet rewarding workout from home, the office, gym, dance studio—or anywhere. Listen to your body and push yourself to continually improve. Remember: **"If it doesn't challenge you, it doesn't change you."**

LEG LIFTS STRAIGHT FORWARD

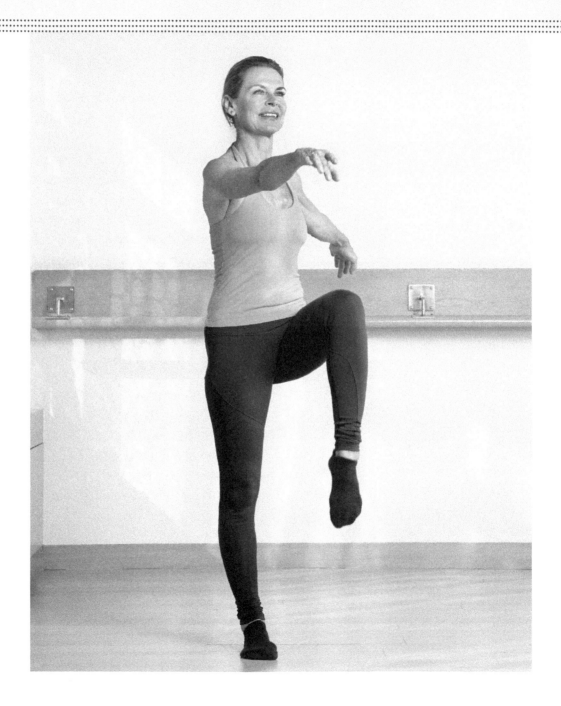

PRIMARY MUSCLES: The rectus femoris and hip flexor muscles lift the knee. The hamstrings, gluteals, and lower back muscles stretch it. The arms swing gently front to back in opposition to the lifting legs.

STABILIZING MUSCLES: The anterior core, which includes the abdominals, especially the transversus abdominis, stabilizes. The upper back muscles also stabilize the trunk.

It is very important to warm up the body in order to increase circulation, respiration, and joint lubrication. Taking time to complete your warm-up will make the exercises safer and help you achieve optimal muscular performance. These leg lifts moving straight forward will help start the warm-up process.

SET UP AND BASIC VARIATION

1. Stand with your feet hip-width apart and parallel.
2. Keep your shoulders down and level. Keep your ears over your shoulders and your shoulders over your hips.
3. Distribute your weight evenly over your feet.
4. Lift your knee below your waist with your heel under your knee and your legs hip-width apart while simultaneously swinging your arms in opposition by your sides.
5. Your arms should swing slightly higher than your shoulder.
6. Keep your standing leg straight.
7. Keep your abdominals pulled in.
8. Lift each leg 15 times.

WATCH OUT FOR
• *Knees lifting too low*

FIX IT
• *Slow your movement down and hold your hand a little higher than your waist to give you a target for proper knee height.*

WATCH OUT FOR
• *Arms too low*

FIX IT
• *Encourage a bigger range of motion for your arms.*

WATCH OUT FOR
• *Moving same side arm as leg*

FIX IT
• *Think of how you normally walk, with your arms swinging in opposition to your lifting leg.*

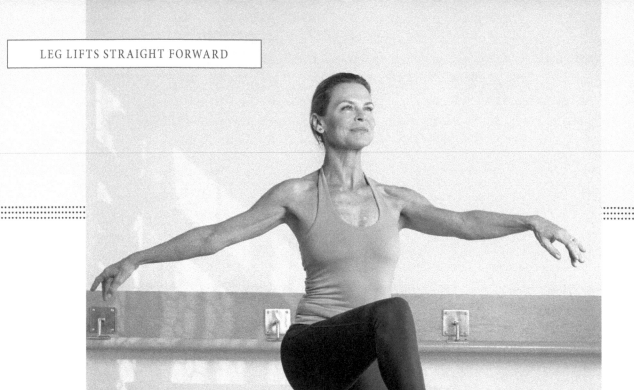

NEXT LEVEL

1. Perform the Set Up and Basic Variation.
2. Lift your knees to your chest.
3. Lift each leg 15 times.

LEG LIFTS WITH GOALPOST ARMS

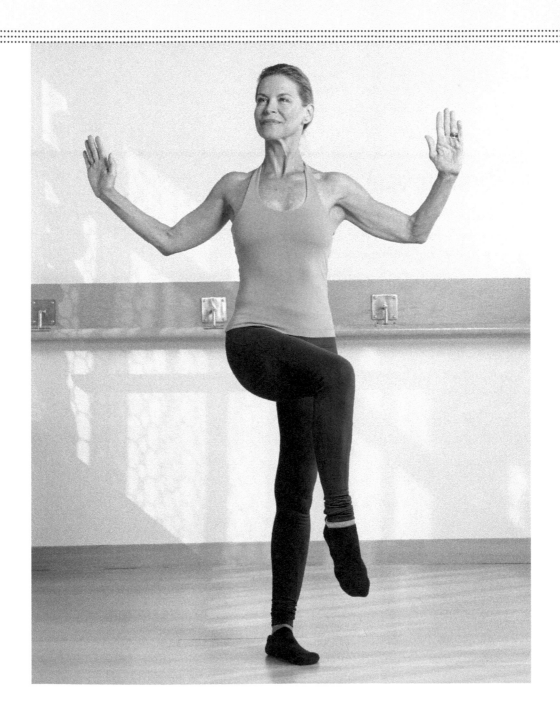

PRIMARY MUSCLES: The rectus femoris and hip flexor muscles lift the knee. The hamstrings, gluteals, and lower back muscles stretch. The arms swing gently front to back in opposition to the lifting leg. The obliques are being warmed up and stretched as the body rotates from side to side to the lifting legs.

STABILIZING MUSCLES: The anterior core—which includes the abdominals, especially the transversus abdominis—helps to stabilize. The upper back muscle group also stabilizes the trunk.

This part of the warm-up will address the rotation or twisting movement of the spine to the right and left and begins to warm up the obliques of the core.

SET UP AND BASIC VARIATION

1. Stand with your feet hip-width apart and parallel.
2. Keep your shoulders down and level. Keep your ears over your shoulders and your shoulders over your hips.
3. Distribute your weight evenly over your feet.
4. Lift your knee below your waist with your heel under your knee and your legs hip-width apart while your arms lift to the goalposts. Keep your arms L-shaped and below shoulder height.
5. Cross your opposite elbow below shoulder height toward your knee, keeping your knee below your waist.
6. Keep your standing leg straight.
7. Keep your abdominals pulled in.
8. Lift each knee 15 times.

WATCH OUT FOR
- *Knees lifting too low*

FIX IT
- *Slow your movement down and hold your hands a little higher than your waist to give you a target for proper knee height.*

WATCH OUT FOR
- *Arms too low*

FIX IT
- *Your elbows should remain at shoulder height as you twist.*

WATCH OUT FOR
- *Small twist*

FIX IT
- *Twist your lifting knee more to your opposite elbow.*

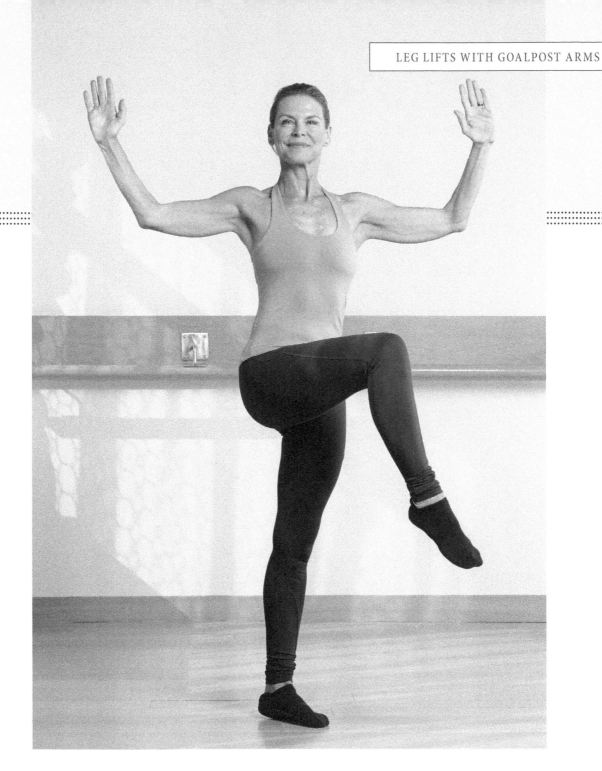

NEXT LEVEL

1. Perform the Set Up and Basic Variation.
2. Lift your knee to your chest and bring your elbows to shoulder height.
3. Lift each knee 15 times.

SECOND POSITION SIDE BEND

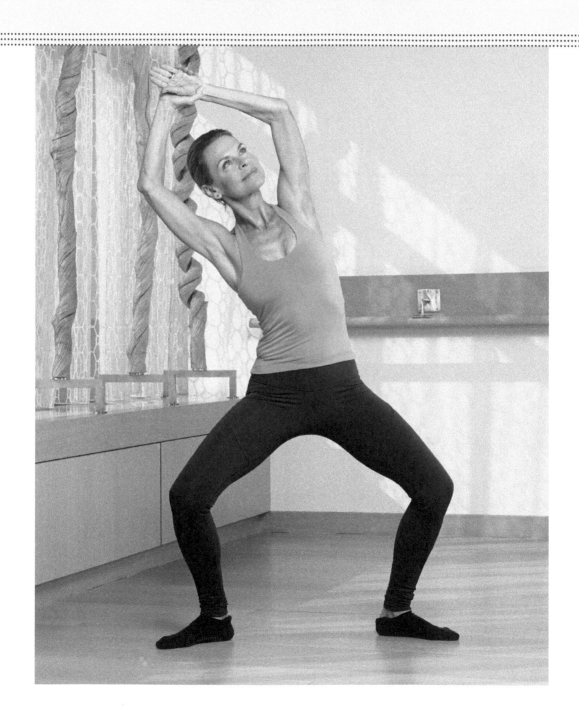

PRIMARY MUSCLES: The quadriceps, gluteus maximus, minimus, medius, and hip abductors and adductors are the primary muscles used in this exercise.

STABILIZING MUSCLES: The abdominals, gluteals, shoulder girdle, and foot muscles will provide stability.

This part of the warm-up helps to achieve lateral flexion of the spine, or side bending. It helps with your breathing as well because it opens up your lungs. This second position also prepares your legs for the thigh-strengthening series.

SET UP AND BASIC VARIATION

1. Step your feet apart into a wide second position with your heels on the ground, keeping your hips above your knees and initiating a turn out from your hips. Your legs should be apart and wider than your hips.

2. Maintain a neutral spine and pull your abdominals in.

3. Keep your shoulders pressed down and level. Keep your ears over your shoulders and your shoulders over your hips.

4. Bend your knees over your feet and keep your hips above your knees.

5. Your feet remain flat on the floor with your weight distributed evenly over them.

6. Reach your arms straight above your shoulders with your palms facing each other and grab your wrist.

7. On an inhale, reach your arms up, straighten your legs, and bend to the right, bending your knees on an exhale.

8. Repeat to the left.

9. Straighten your knees on the way up and soften them on the side bend.

10. Repeat 4 times.

NOTE

Wide second position is a stance where your feet are wider than hip-width apart in a V shape. Your feet are flat on the floor. The turn-out happens from the hips.

WATCH OUT FOR
• *Pelvis tips back*

FIX IT
• *Use your gluteus more in a forward position, pull your abdominals in, and elongate through your spine.*

WATCH OUT FOR
• *Too turned out from the ankles and feet*

FIX IT
• *Place each foot more at a 45-degree angle, so your hip, knee, foot are stacked on top of each other.*

WATCH OUT FOR
• *Leaning forward in upper body*

FIX IT
• *Press your shoulders down and back and engage your abdominals more.*

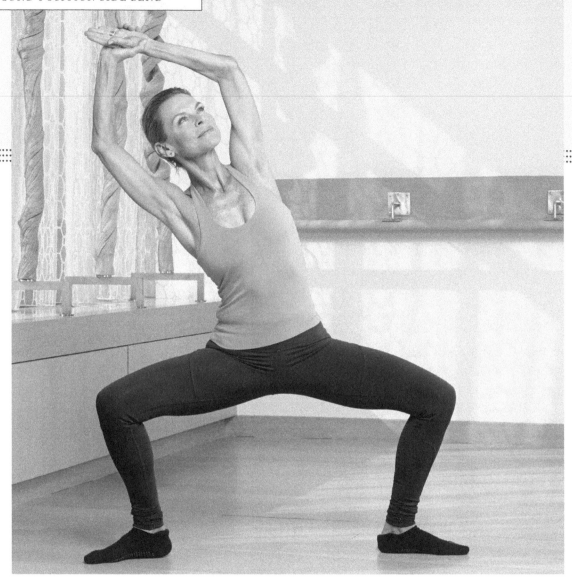

NEXT LEVEL

1. Perform the Set Up and Basic Variation.
2. Bring your hips to knee level.
3. Repeat 4 times.

NOTE

A **neutral spine** refers to the natural curves of the spine—cervical, thoracic, lumbar, and sacral. Ideal posture indicates proper alignment of the body's segments, resulting in the least amount of stress placed on the body's tissues. In this position, you are able to completely and optimally attain balance and proportion of your body mass and framework, based on your physical limitations. Good posture optimizes breathing and assists the circulation of body fluids.

>Warm-Up<
SECOND POSITION PLIÉS

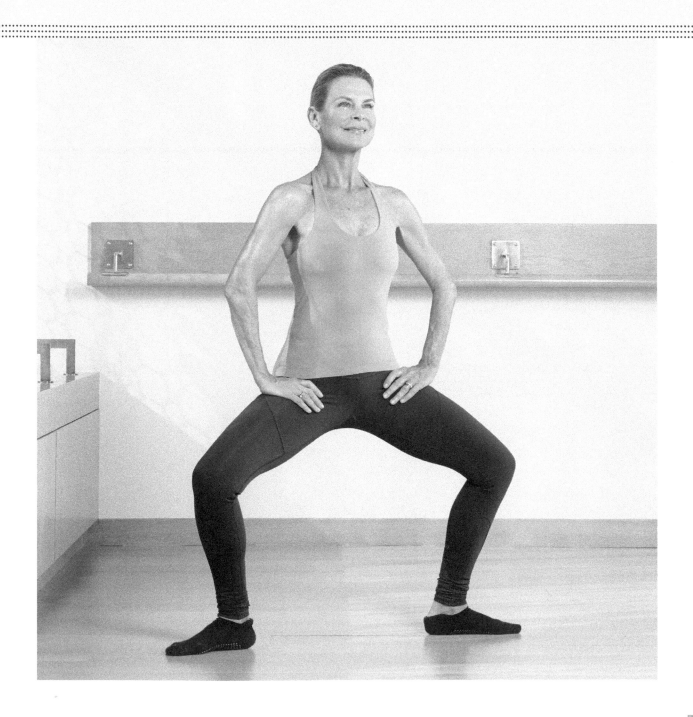

PRIMARY MUSCLES: The quadriceps, gluteus maximus, minimus, medius, and hip abductors and adductors are the primary muscles used in this exercise.

STABILIZING MUSCLES: The abdominals, gluteals, shoulder girdle, and foot muscles help to stabilize.

This section of the warm-up helps to prepare the legs for the thigh-strengthening section of the book. It also warms up the hips and knees for all the turn out and parallel leg positions. This allows for better joint lubrication and increased blood flow.

SET UP AND BASIC VARIATION

1. Drop your tailbone to a neutral spine and pull your abdominals in.
2. Keep your shoulders pressed down and level. Keep your ears over your shoulders and your shoulders over your hips.
3. Open your legs and separate your feet so they are wider than hip-width apart.
4. Keep your hips, knees, and feet aligned on top of each other. Keep even weight distribution over your feet.
5. Bend your knees over your feet, initiating a turn out from your hips.
6. Keep your feet flat on the floor.
7. With a straight back, lower your body, keeping your hips above your knees. Keep your abdominals pulled in.
8. Bend and straighten your legs down and up a couple of inches (5 cm) with your hands on your hips and with your hips always remaining above knee level. Perform 8 times.
9. Keep your hands on your hips, which should be a few inches (7 to 10 cm) above knee level, and pulse 8 times.

WATCH OUT FOR
- *Pelvis tips back*

FIX IT
- *Use your gluteus more in the forward position, pull your abdominals in, and elongate through your spine.*

WATCH OUT FOR
- *Too turned out from the ankles and feet*

FIX IT
- *Place each foot more at a 45-degree angle, so your hip, knee, and foot are stacked on top of each other.*

WATCH OUT FOR
- *Leaning forward in upper body*

FIX IT
- *Press your shoulders down and back and engage your abdominals more.*

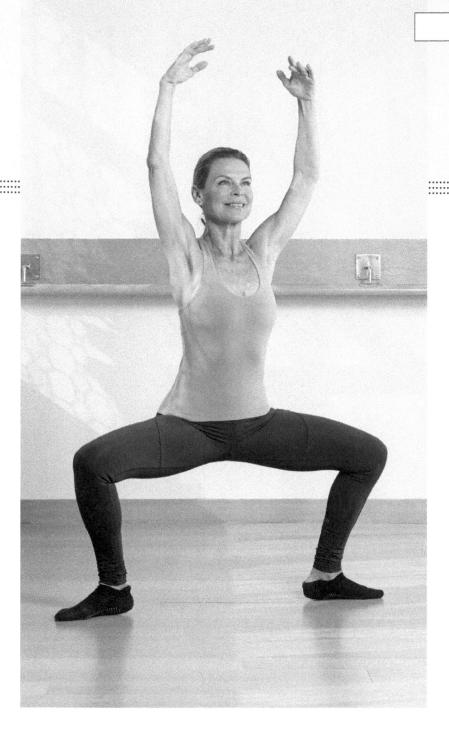

NEXT LEVEL

1. Perform the Set Up and Basic Variation.

2. With a straight back, lower your body, bringing your hips to knee level. Keep your abdominals pulled in.

3. As your hips reach knee level, raise your arms straight out to the side and up above your shoulders; then straighten your legs as you move your arms down to the side and in front of your hips. Perform 8 times.

4. Lower your body so your hips are at knee level with your arms up above your shoulders. Pulse 8 times.

NOTE

A **plié** is a movement in which a dancer bends the knees and straightens them again, usually with the hips turned out and the heels pressed together.

SECOND POSITION PLIÉ WITH BALANCE

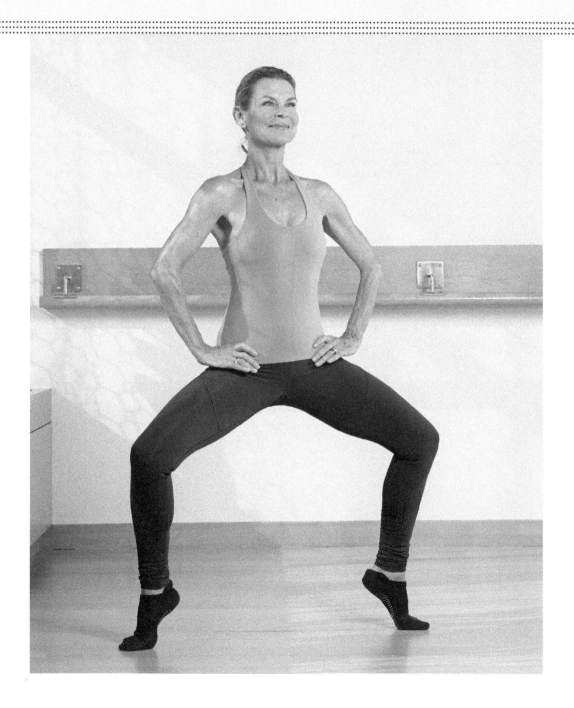

PRIMARY MUSCLES: The quadriceps, gluteus maximus, minimus, medius, hip abductors and adductors, and gastrocnemius are the primary muscles used in this exercise.

STABILIZING MUSCLES: The abdominals, gluteals, shoulder girdle, and foot muscles provide stability.

This part of the warm-up helps to create a sense of balance and to warm up the feet and legs for the thigh-strengthening section.

SET UP AND BASIC VARIATION

1. Drop your tailbone to a neutral spine and pull in your abdominals.

2. Keep your shoulders pressed down and level. Keep your ears over your shoulders and your shoulders over your hips.

3. Open your legs and separate your feet so they are wider than hip-width apart.

4. Keep your hips, knees, and feet aligned on top of each other. Distribute your weight evenly over your feet.

5. Place your hands on your hips with your shoulders pressing down and back.

6. Bend your knees over your feet and turn out from the hips.

7. Raise your heels and balance on the balls of your feet.

8. Keep your hips above your knees. Keep your abdominals pulled in.

9. Balance 4 counts and then straighten your legs.

WATCH OUT FOR
- *Pelvis tips back*

FIX IT
- *Use your gluteus more in a forward position, pull your abdominals in, and elongate through your spine.*

WATCH OUT FOR
- *Turned out too much from the ankles and feet*

FIX IT
- *Place each foot more at a 45-degree angle, so your hip, knee, and foot are stacked on top of each other.*

WATCH OUT FOR
- *Upper body leaning forward*

FIX IT
- *Press your shoulders down and back and engage your abdominals more.*

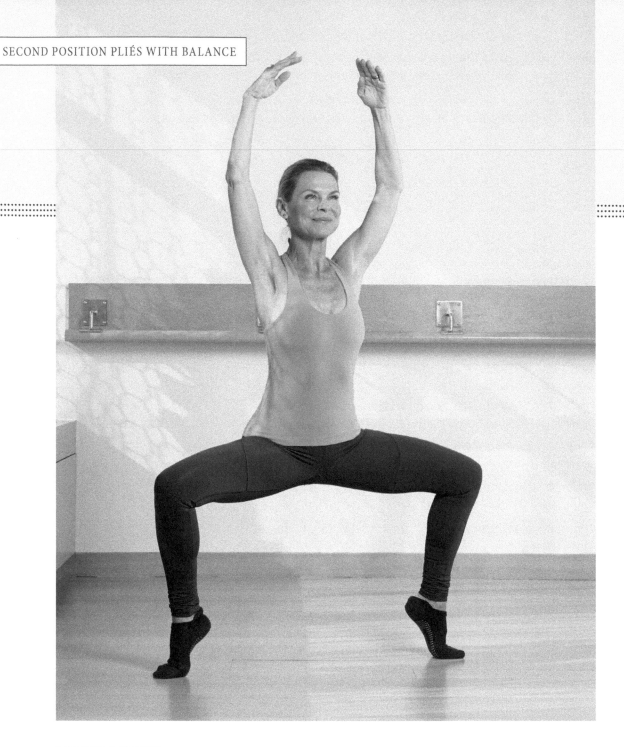

NEXT LEVEL

1. Perform the Set Up and Basic Variation.

2. Raise one heel off the floor onto the ball of your foot, then the other, so both heels come off the floor.

3. Balance 4 counts and then straighten your legs.

BACK BEND

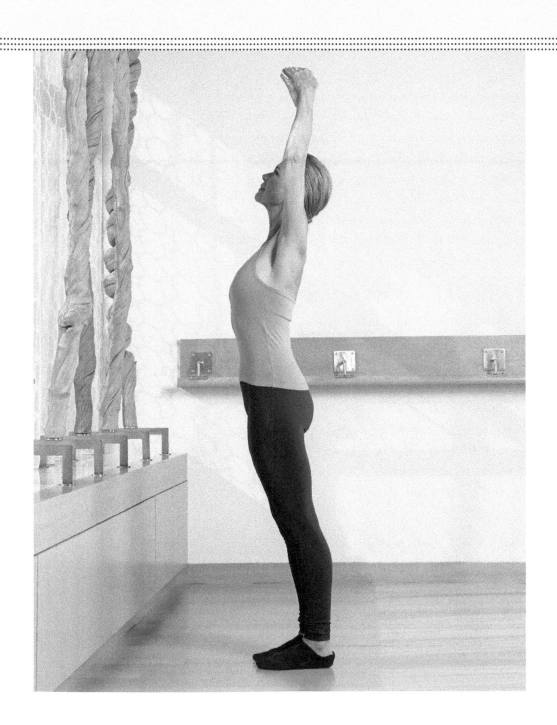

PRIMARY MUSCLES: The gluteus maximus and back extensor muscles are the primary muscles used in this exercise.

STABILIZING MUSCLES: The gluteals, abdominals, and foot muscles provide stability.

This back bend section of the warm-up prepares the spine for extension movement, or arching. It starts to strengthen the back muscles, enabling the synovial fluid to lubricate the joints of the vertebrae. The final section of the warm-up prepares the spine for flexion movement, or forward folding of the body. The forward fold also targets the hamstrings to prepare them for flexibility and stretches the back muscles. Forward folding helps to focus your mind because this type of movement is very introspective.

SET UP AND BASIC VARIATION

1. Keep a neutral spine and pull in your abdominals.

2. Keep your shoulders pressed down and level.

3. Keep your ears over your shoulders with the bottom of your chin parallel to the floor.

4. Your feet should be hip-width apart and parallel.

5. Your hips, knees, and feet should be aligned parallel over each other. Distribute your weight evenly over your feet.

6. Soften your knees over your feet.

7. Keep your feet flat on the floor.

8. Keep your abdominals pulled in.

9. Reach your arms up straight above your shoulders with your palms facing each other on the inhale. Arch your back from the lower back with a **minimal back bend** on the exhale while the rest of the spine follows the extension from your lower back.

WATCH OUT FOR
- *Pelvis tips forward too much, sinking body weight into lower back*

FIX IT
- *Soften your knees more to engage your quadriceps for foundation stability, pull your abdominals in, and elongate through your spine before arching your back.*

WATCH OUT FOR
- *Turned out too much from the ankles and feet*

FIX IT
- *Check that your hips, knees, and feet are stacked on top of each other.*

WATCH OUT FOR
- *Head drops back too far*

FIX IT
- *Bring your chin more toward your throat and keep the natural cervical spine curve. The spinal extension begins from your lower back lumbar spine and travels upward to your thoracic and then cervical spine.*

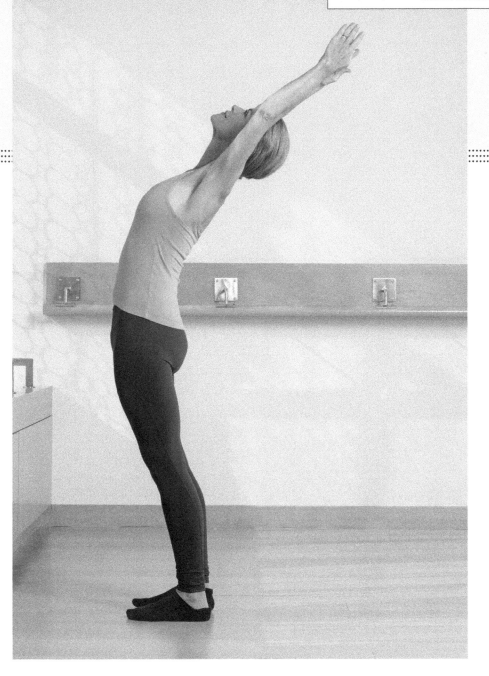

NEXT LEVEL

1. Perform the Set Up and Basic Variation.
2. Keeping your arms straight above your shoulders with your palms facing each other on the inhale, increase the arch from the lower back initiation with a **big back bend** on the exhale. The rest of your spine follows the extension from your lower back.

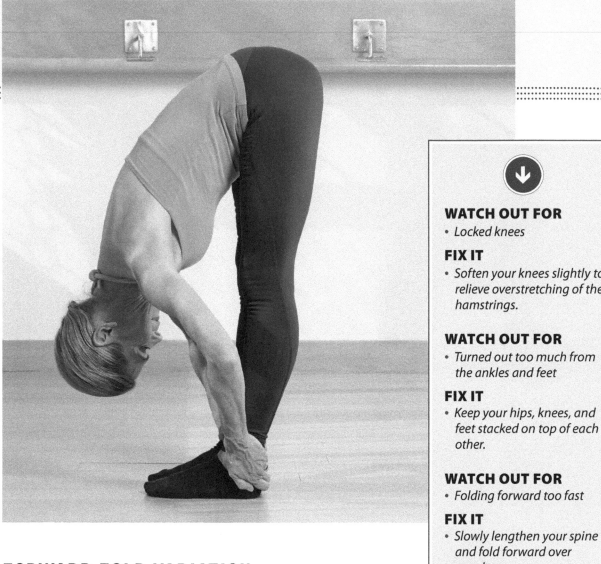

WATCH OUT FOR
- *Locked knees*

FIX IT
- *Soften your knees slightly to relieve overstretching of the hamstrings.*

WATCH OUT FOR
- *Turned out too much from the ankles and feet*

FIX IT
- *Keep your hips, knees, and feet stacked on top of each other.*

WATCH OUT FOR
- *Folding forward too fast*

FIX IT
- *Slowly lengthen your spine and fold forward over your legs.*

FORWARD FOLD VARIATION

1. Perform either version of the back bend.
2. On an exhale, fold forward from your hips with a flat back, reaching your hands onto your ankles or shins. Bend your knees slightly, if necessary.
3. Your spine is lengthened naturally forward, initiating from your hips, lumbar, thoracic, and cervical spine.

FOREARM PLANK

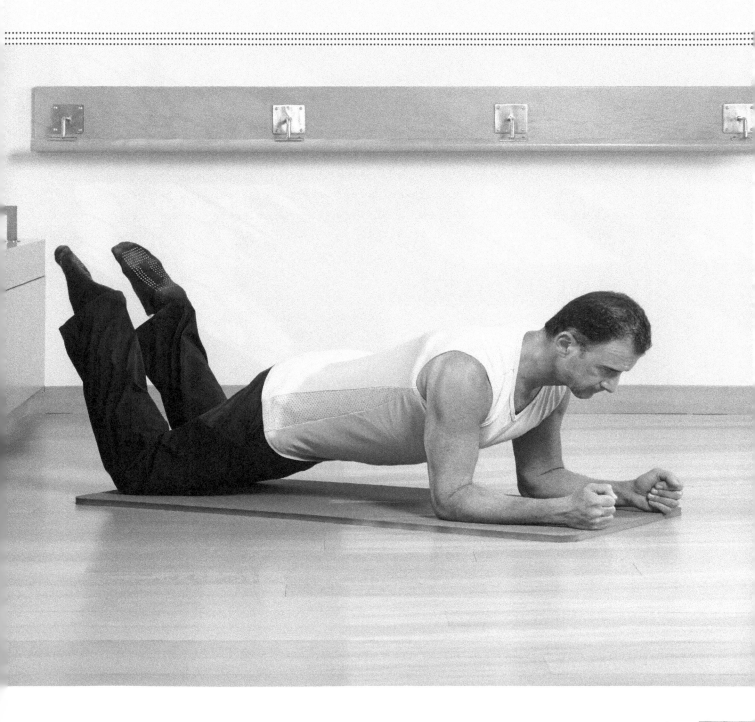

PRIMARY MUSCLES: The abdominals, especially the transversus abdominis, deltoids, pectorals, and biceps are the primary muscles used in this exercise.

STABILIZING MUSCLES: The abdominal muscles provide stability.

Though this book has quite a lot of lower body exercises, you also need to balance with upper body work. Planks are ideal for building core strength, and the forearm plank adds upper body focus as well as trunk strength and stabilization. Also, the plank reference, that feeling of holding your abdominal muscles in toward your spine, needs to be constant throughout all your upper and lower body exercises. Other movements depend on a stable, solid core. How long can you hold a plank?

SET UP AND BASIC VARIATION

1. Place your forearms down on the floor, shoulder-width apart (elbows under your shoulders) and parallel. Keep your wrists parallel to each other with the palm side of your fists facing each other.

2. Press your shoulders away from your ears.

3. Begin with your legs bent and place your lower front thigh on the floor, taking the weight off your knees.

4. Engage your abdominals by pulling in. (Emphasize the abdominal lock and breathing without moving your abdominals.)

5. Press your shoulders down and lengthen your neck.

6. Check for spine alignment, proper head alignment, and observe that your hips stay in line with your shoulders.

7. Hold for 30 seconds, building up to 60 seconds. Your goal is to increase your duration.

WATCH OUT FOR
• *Back arching*

FIX IT
• *Drop to your knees and reaffirm your abdominals.*

WATCH OUT FOR
• *Head hanging*

FIX IT
• *Bring your chin in and keep your ears in line with your shoulders.*

WATCH OUT FOR
• *Hips rising or sinking*

FIX IT
• *Maintain your ears in line with your shoulders, your shoulders in line with your hips, and your hips in line with your heels if your legs are straight.*

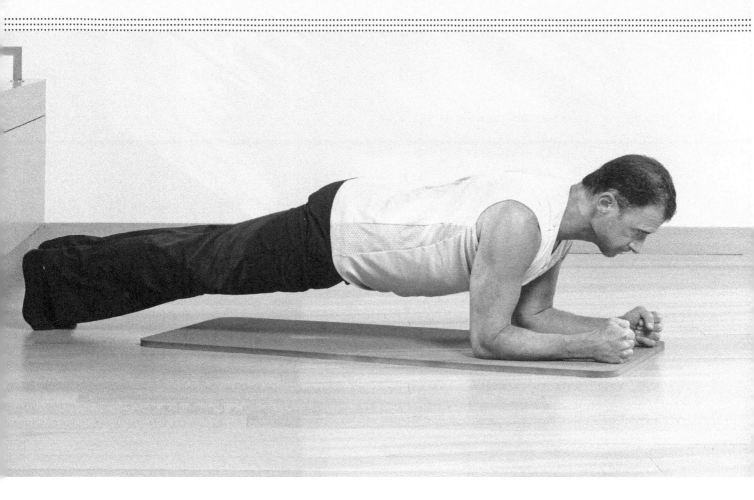

STRAIGHT LEG VARIATION

1. Perform the Set Up and Basic Variation.

2. Lift your knees off the floor, engage your thighs, and lengthen through your heels.

3. Hold for 30 seconds, building up to 60 seconds. Your goal is to increase your duration.

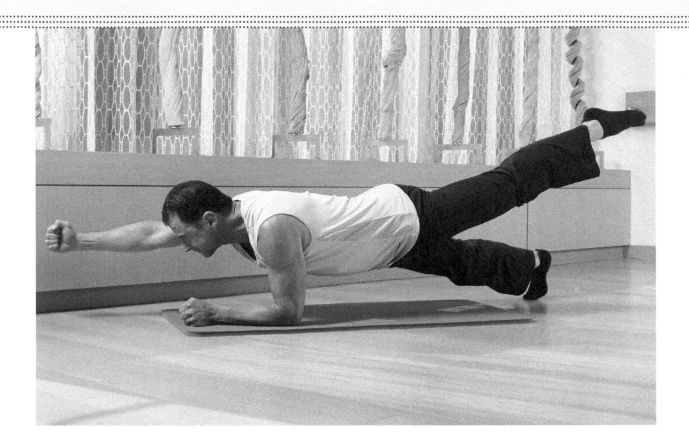

ADVANCED VARIATION

1. Perform the Set Up and Basic Variation.

2. Extend your right arm and left leg off the floor.

3. Hold for 15 seconds.

4. Repeat with the other arm and leg off the floor.

5. Hold for 15 seconds. Your goal is to increase your duration.

SIDE ARM PLANK

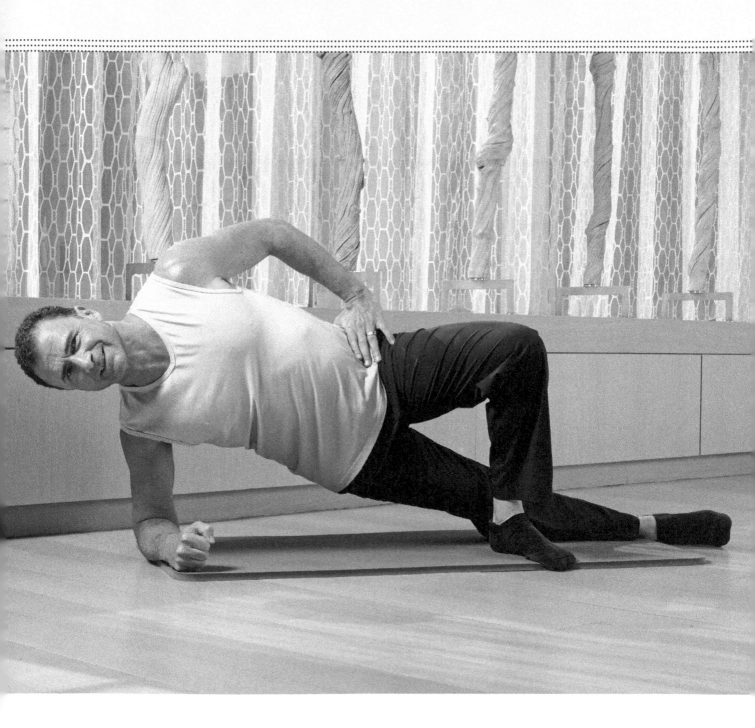

PRIMARY MUSCLES: The abdominals, especially the transverse abdominis and internal and external obliques, shoulder girdle, and arms are the primary muscles used in this exercise.

STABILIZING MUSCLES: The abdominals, shoulder girdle, and pelvic floor provide stability.

The Side Arm Plank will help you achieve more trunk/abdominal strength and stabilization with a focus on the internal and external obliques. You'll gain upper-body strength and endurance—especially as you gradually increase the amount of time you can hold a plank.

SET UP AND BASIC VARIATION

1. Make a fist with both hands.
2. Take your right-hand fist to your left elbow and place your right elbow under your right shoulder with your right arm making an L-shape.
3. Turn on to the outside edge of your right foot.
4. Keep your hips stacked over each other with your legs straight and your feet flexed.
5. Step with a bent left leg in front of your right bottom straight leg. Your left foot should be flat on the floor.
6. Keep your ears over your shoulders and your shoulders over your hips. Keep your chin parallel to the floor.
7. Keep your hips, knees, and ankles stacked on top of each other.
8. Keep your body weight on the outside edge of the right foot.
9. With your shoulders stacked on top of each other, reach your top arm straight over your ear/above your shoulder with your palm down.
10. Keep your abdominals pulled in and your shoulders pressed down.
11. Hold for 10 to 15 seconds.
12. Repeat on the other side.

WATCH OUT FOR
- *Back arching*

FIX IT
- *Step down your top foot and place with your knee bent in front of your bottom foot. Reaffirm your abdominals.*

WATCH OUT FOR
- *Head hanging*

FIX IT
- *Bring your chin in and keep your ears in line with your shoulders.*

WATCH OUT FOR
- *Hips rising or sinking*

FIX IT
- *Keep your ears in line with your shoulders, your shoulders in line with your hips, and your hips in line with your heels if your legs are straight.*

WATCH OUT FOR
- *Pelvis dropping*

FIX IT
- *Keep your hips in line with your shoulders.*

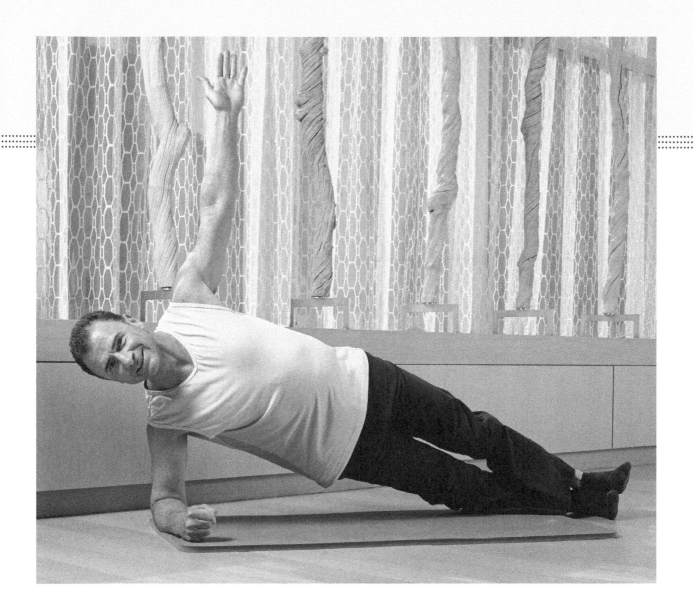

STRAIGHT LEG VARIATION

1. Perform the Set Up and Basic Variation.
2. Keep your hips stacked over each other with both legs straight and your feet flexed.
3. Hold for 10 to 15 seconds.
4. Repeat on the other side.

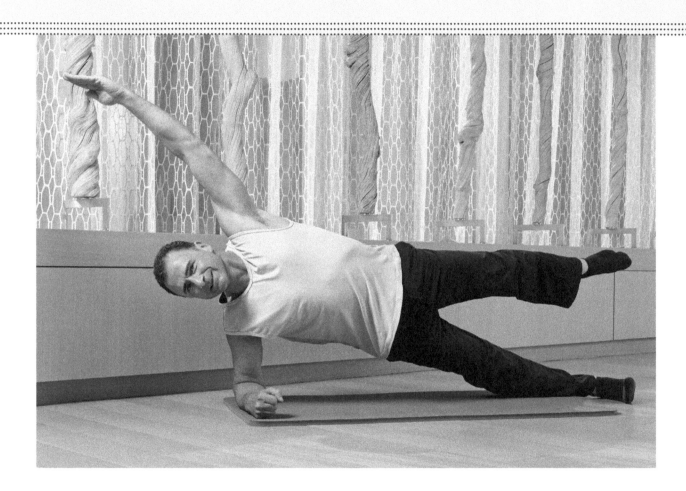

ADVANCED

1. Perform the Set Up and Basic Variation and the Next Level.

2. Raise your right leg straight off your left leg.

3. Hold for 10 seconds.

4. Repeat on the other side.

FRONT PECTORAL PUSH-UPS

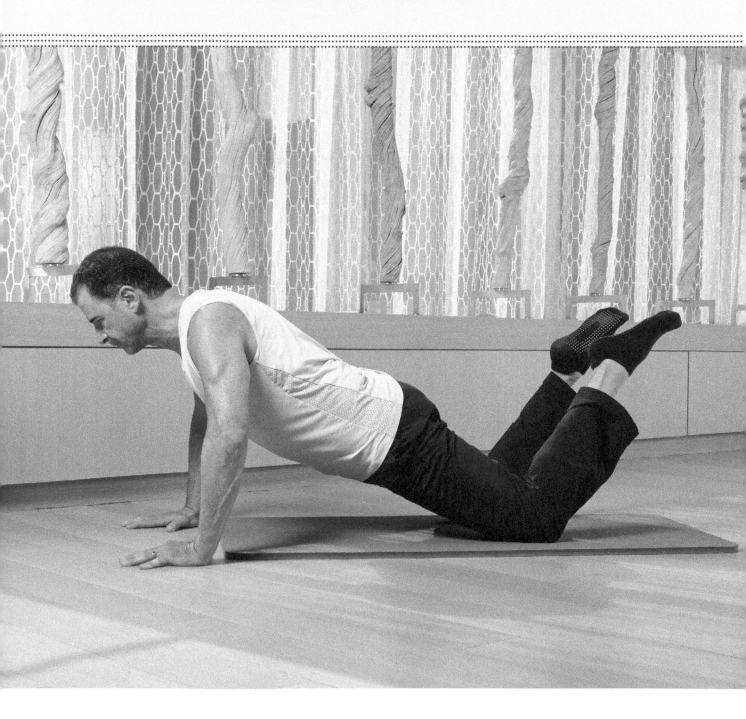

PRIMARY MUSCLES: The pectorals, biceps, deltoids, triceps, trapezius, and teres major/minor are the primary muscles used in this exercise.

STABILIZING MUSCLES: The abdominals and neck extensors provide stability.

These push-ups will help strengthen the entire upper body musculature, including the chest, back, and arms. This exercise is also a weight-bearing exercise. It is best to think of this exercise as a moving plank.

SET UP AND BASIC VARIATION

1. Place your hands (with your fingers spread open and facing mostly forward) off the mat a bit wider than your shoulders on the floor.

2. Shift your weight to the front of your thighs with your bent knees slightly wider than your hips and your feet uncrossed and toward your gluteals.

3. Assume a horizontal body position with your ears over your shoulders, your chin in, your tailbone dropped, your shoulders over your hips and your fingers spread open.

4. Lower your body a couple of inches or midway down (5 cm) and lift along a horizontal line.

5. Slowly do 10 push-ups.

6. Do 10 more push-ups a little faster.

7. Soften your elbows and hold for 10 seconds.

8. Perform a child's pose with both arms extended forward.

WATCH OUT FOR
- *Neck arching*

FIX IT
- *Keep your chin toward your throat and your ears over your shoulders. Lead with your chest. Fix your eyes slightly forward.*

WATCH OUT FOR
- *Back arching*

FIX IT
- *Drop to your knees and reaffirm your abdominals, pulling them in toward your spine. Stay higher on the lowering movement.*

WATCH OUT FOR
- *Hips rising or sinking*

FIX IT
- *Maintain your ears in line with your shoulders, your shoulders in line with your hips, and your hips in line with your heels if your legs are straight.*

WATCH OUT FOR
- *Shoulder discomfort*

FIX IT
- *Keep your hands under your shoulders or do the standing push-up at a barre or wall.*

WATCH OUT FOR
- *Wrist discomfort*

FIX IT
- *Make a fist with your hands, bend your knees, minimize the lowering, or do the standing push-up at a barre or wall.*

WATCH OUT FOR
- *Elbows locking*

FIX IT
- *Always keep a slight bend in your elbows on the extension.*

WATCH OUT FOR
- *Head hanging*

FIX IT
- *Keep your ears in line with your shoulders.*

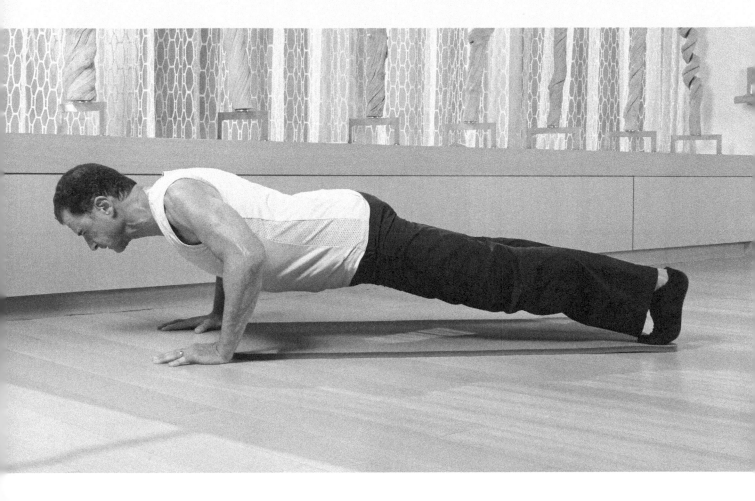

NEXT LEVEL

1. Perform the Set Up and Basic Variation.

2. With your feet slightly wider than your hips, tuck your toes under and straighten both legs.

3. Your body should be lowered about midway to the floor and lifted along a horizontal line.

4. Slowly do 10 push-ups.

5. Do 10 more push-ups a little faster.

6. Soften into your elbows and hold for 10 seconds.

7. Assume a child's pose with both arms extended forward.

NOTE

Child's pose (page 140) is a position in which you sit on your heels with your feet together, your knees open, and your upper body folded forward down the center.

REVERSE PUSH-UP

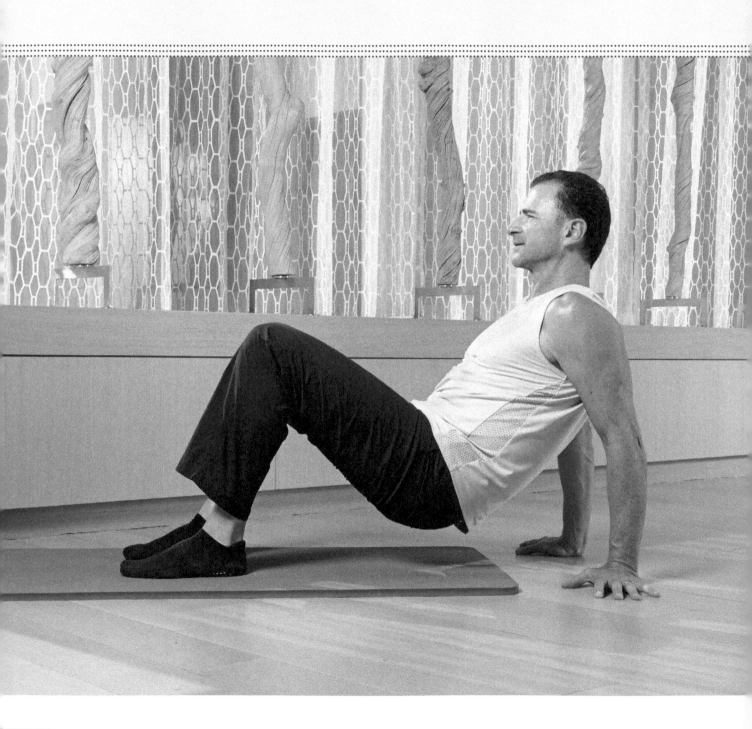

PRIMARY MUSCLES: The triceps, anconueus, posterior deltoid, and all other arm extensors are the primary muscles used in this exercise.

STABILIZING MUSCLES: The abdominals, levator scapuli, and inferior shoulder girdle muscles provide stability.

This push-up builds strength and definition in the back of the arm (triceps primarily) and shoulder region while also engaging the abdominals. It is also considered a weight-bearing exercise because you are lifting and lowering your body against gravity.

SET UP AND BASIC VARIATION

1. Sitting on the floor, bend your knees in front of your hips at a right 90-degree angle. Keep your feet flat on the floor.

2. Place your hands slightly behind your shoulders, a little wider than shoulder width with your thumbs parallel to each other facing toward your hips and your fingers spread open, pressing your thumbs and fingers into the floor.

3. Shift your body weight back into your arms.

4. Keep your ears over your shoulders and your shoulders rolled down and back.

5. Keep your gaze forward (not upward).

6. Keep your abdominals pulled in.

7. With your gluteals on the floor, bend and straighten your elbows 10 to 15 times, keeping a slight bend in your elbows on the extension.

8. Tuck your gluteals up and raise your hips off the floor at least 12 inches (30.5 cm). Shift your body weight back into your arms and hands.

9. Bend and straighten your elbows 10 to 15 times, keeping a slight bend in your elbows on the extension. Avoid your hips dropping or sagging.

WATCH OUT FOR
- *Elbows locking*

FIX IT
- *Reduce the number of repetitions and use only the bent-leg variation. Always keep a slight bend in your elbows on the extension.*

WATCH OUT FOR
- *Strain in hands or wrist*

FIX IT
- *Check your hand foundation and spread out your fingers. Keep your gluteals on the floor. Bend and extend your elbows while sitting to minimize the weight in your hands. Or make fists with your hands and put your weight on your knuckles with your flat wrist.*

WATCH OUT FOR
- *Shoulders riding up when elbows bend*

FIX IT
- *Rotate your shoulders down more. Use the bent leg variation and fewer reps.*

WATCH OUT FOR
- *Hips dip instead of elbows bending*

FIX IT
- *Keep your hips lifted and initiate the bend from your elbows.*

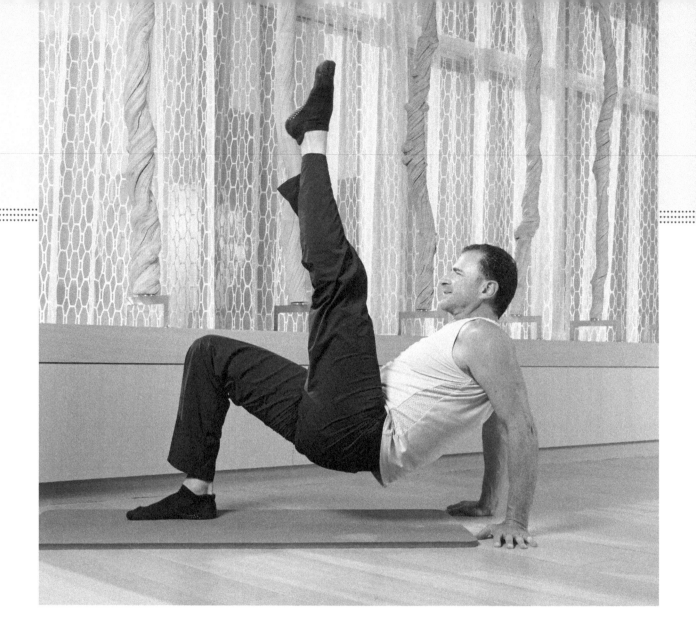

ONE-LEG VARIATION

1. Perform the Set Up and Basic Variation.

2. Keep one knee bent with your foot flat on the floor and your opposite leg extended perpendicular to the floor above your hip with your foot pointed.

3. The heel of your extended leg must be over your hip. If this is inaccessible, bend your knee instead and place your foot above your knee on the thigh of the bottom supporting leg.

4. Bend and straighten your elbows 10 times, keeping a slight bend in your elbows on the extension. Avoid your hips dropping or sagging.

5. Repeat with your other leg.

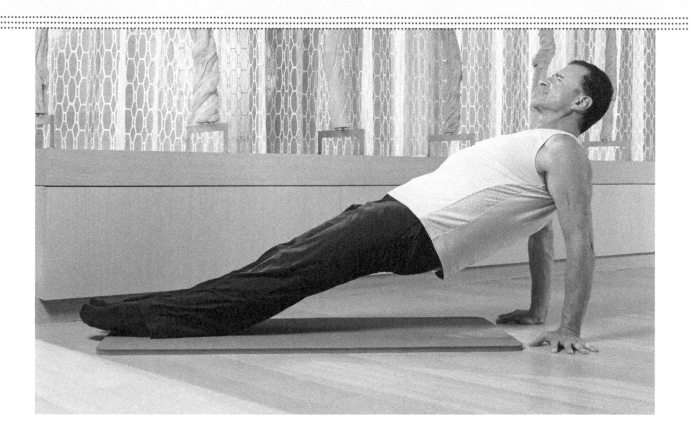

BOTH LEGS STRAIGHT VARIATION

1. Perform the Set Up and Basic Variation and the One-Leg Variation.

2. Extend both legs straight (parallel or turned out) directly out in front of your hips with your feet pointed.

3. Press your pelvis up so your hips are flat and in line with your shoulders.

4. Bend and straighten your elbows 10 times, keeping a slight bend in your elbows on the extension. Keep your hips from dropping or sagging.

DELTOID PRESS

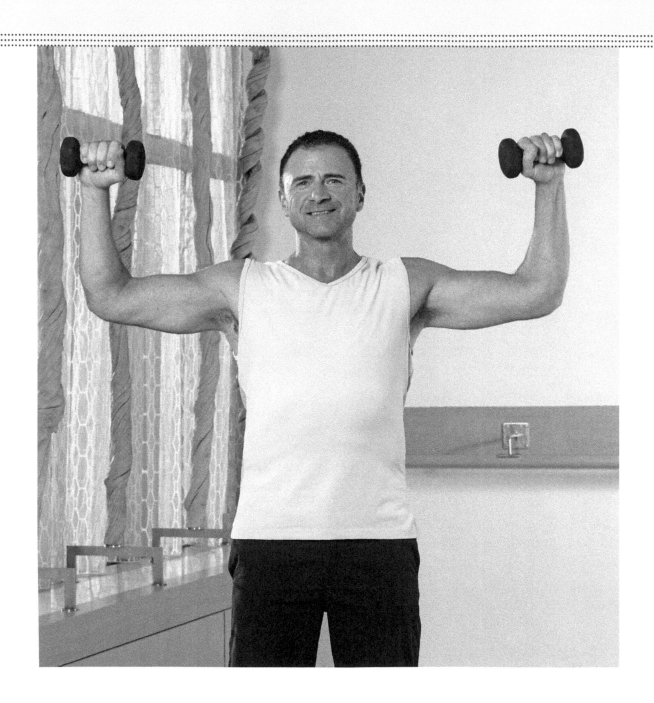

PRIMARY MUSCLES: In the pull-down phase, the latissimus dorsi and upper back muscles are used primarily; in the push-up phase, the deltoid and the biceps are used.

STABILIZING MUSCLES: The abdominals, gluteals, and thighs provide stability.

This exercise uses 2- to 5-pound (1 to 2.5 kg) weights to help build a balance of strength and range of motion in the shoulder girdle, which will help maintain proper posture of the upper body and avoid the forward rounding of shoulders. This will give you a dancer's posture.

SET UP AND BASIC VARIATION

1. Stand with your feet hip-width apart and parallel.
2. Soften your knees.
3. With 2- to 5-pound (1 to 2.5 kg) hand weights, depending on your level, wrap all your fingers evenly around the stem of the weight.
4. Keep your ears/shoulders/hips stacked on top of each other with even weight distribution over your feet.
5. Keep a neutral spine and your abdominals engaged.
6. Bend your arms to 90 degrees.
7. Bring your elbows to shoulder height, your hands above your elbows, and keep your wrists flat with your palms facing forward.

(Continued on next page.)

WATCH OUT FOR
- *Back arching*

FIX IT
- *Drop your tailbone and reaffirm your abdominals.*

WATCH OUT FOR
- *Hands falling forward*

FIX IT
- *Rotate your elbows forward and your hands back. A lighter weight or no weights may be needed.*

WATCH OUT FOR
- *Head drops or chin lifts and juts forward*

FIX IT
- *Look straight ahead, and level your chin to be parallel to the floor. Maintain your ears over your shoulders.*

WATCH OUT FOR
- *Hands too high (tapping weights over head instead of in front of forehead)*

FIX IT
- *Bring the weights forward.*

WATCH OUT FOR
- *Wrists bending toward forearm*

FIX IT
- *Flatten your wrist and bring your knuckles over your wrist.*

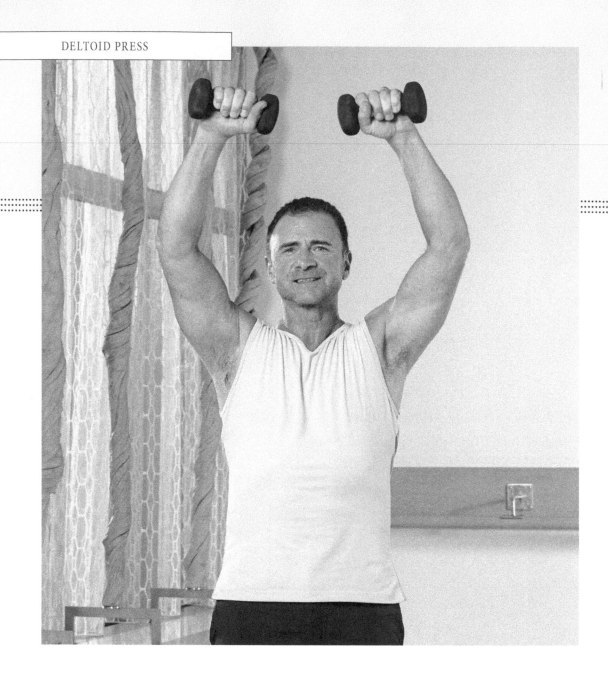

8. Begin to press your arms above your shoulders with your hands slightly in front of your forehead and an exhale on the up movement.

9. Bring your elbows back to shoulder height on the inhale.

10. Lift your arms above your shoulders and lower your arms to shoulder height 20 times.

CHEST PRESS

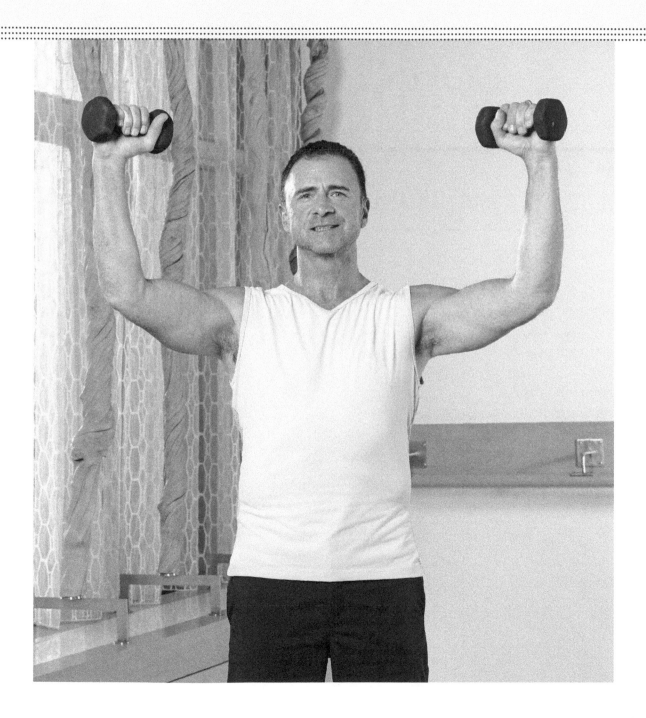

PRIMARY MUSCLES: The pectoralis major and minor, subclavius, anterior and medial deltoids, and biceps are the primary muscles used in this exercise.

STABILIZING MUSCLES: The anterior core/abdominals, thighs and gluteals, and upper back muscular group provide stability.

This exercise uses 2- to 5-pound (1 to 2.5 kg) weights to increase muscular strength and tone in the chest, arms, and shoulders. This will focus on developing the pectoral muscles that help stabilize the front of the shoulders.

SET UP AND BASIC VARIATION

1. Stand with your feet hip-width apart and parallel.
2. Soften your knees.
3. With 2- to 5-pound (1 to 2.5 kg) hand weights, depending on your level, wrap all your fingers evenly around the stem of the weight.
4. Keep your ears/shoulders/hips stacked on top of each other with even weight distribution over your feet.
5. Keep a neutral spine and your abdominals engaged, feeling the plank energy.
6. Bring your elbows to shoulder height in a 90-degree angle. Keep your hands above your elbows and your wrists flat with your palms facing forward.

WATCH OUT FOR
- *Arms coming out of parallel position toward each other when moving*

FIX IT
- *Use less range of motion and keep your wrists over your elbows.*

WATCH OUT FOR
- *Back arching and rocking*

FIX IT
- *Pull in your abdominals and drop your tailbone.*

WATCH OUT FOR
- *Shoulders rising*

FIX IT
- *Settle down your shoulders and use a lighter weight or no weights.*

WATCH OUT FOR
- *Wrists bending back*

FIX IT
- *Keep your hand, wrist, and elbow in one line stacked over each other.*

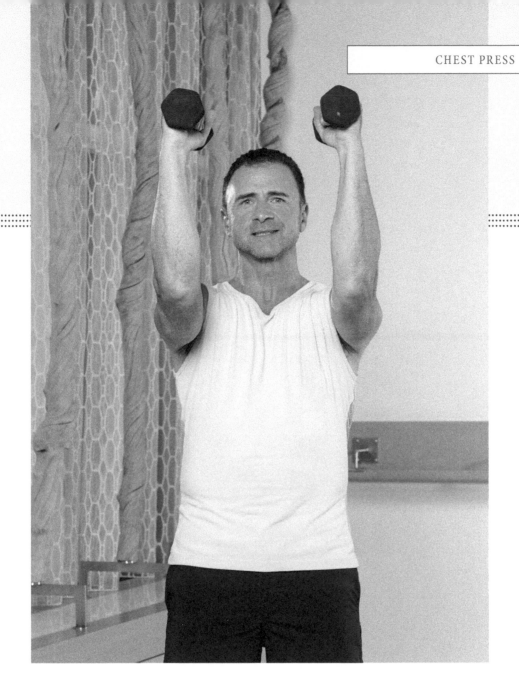

CHEST PRESS

7. On an exhale, keeping your elbows at shoulder height, move your arms toward the center of your body, stopping when your elbows are in front of your shoulders.

8. The heads of the weights face forward.

9. On an inhale, open your arms back to the Set Up position.

10. Repeat 20 times, opening and closing your arms.

VERTICAL PRESS

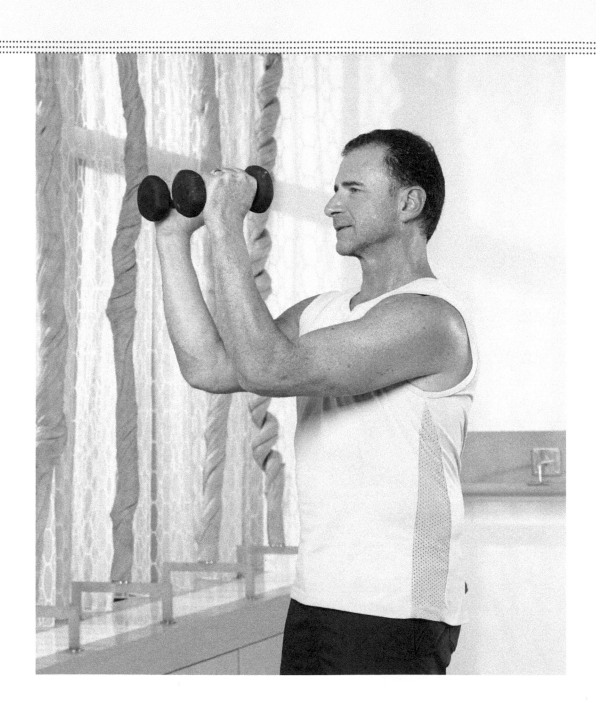

PRIMARY MUSCLES: The pectorals major and minor, subclavius, anterior and medial deltoids, and biceps are the primary muscles used in this exercise.

STABILIZING MUSCLES: The anterior core/abdominals, thighs and gluteals, and upper back muscular group provide stability.

This exercise uses 2- to 5-pound (1 to 2.5 kg) weights to increase muscular strength and tone in the chest, arms, and shoulders. This will focus on developing the pectoral, deltoids, and biceps, muscles that help stabilize the front of the shoulders with very small movements.

SET UP AND BASIC VARIATION

1. Stand with your feet hip-width apart and parallel.

2. Soften your knees.

3. With 2- to 5-pound (1 to 2.5 kg) hand weights, depending on your level, wrap all your fingers evenly around the stem of the weight.

4. Keep your ears/shoulders/hips stacked on top of each other with even weight distribution over your feet.

5. Maintain a neutral spine and keep your abdominals engaged, feeling the plank energy.

6. Bring your elbows to shoulder height in a 90-degree angle directly in front of your shoulders. Your hands stay above your elbows, your wrists are flat, and your palms face each other.

WATCH OUT FOR
- *Arms coming out of parallel position toward each other when moving*

FIX IT
- *Use less range of motion and keep your wrists over your elbows.*

WATCH OUT FOR
- *Back arching and rocking*

FIX IT
- *Pull in your abdominals and drop your tailbone.*

WATCH OUT FOR
- *Shoulders rising*

FIX IT
- *Settle down your shoulders and use a lighter weight or no weights.*

WATCH OUT FOR
- *Wrists bending back*

FIX IT
- *Keep your hand, wrist, and elbow in one line stacked over each other.*

(Continued on next page.)

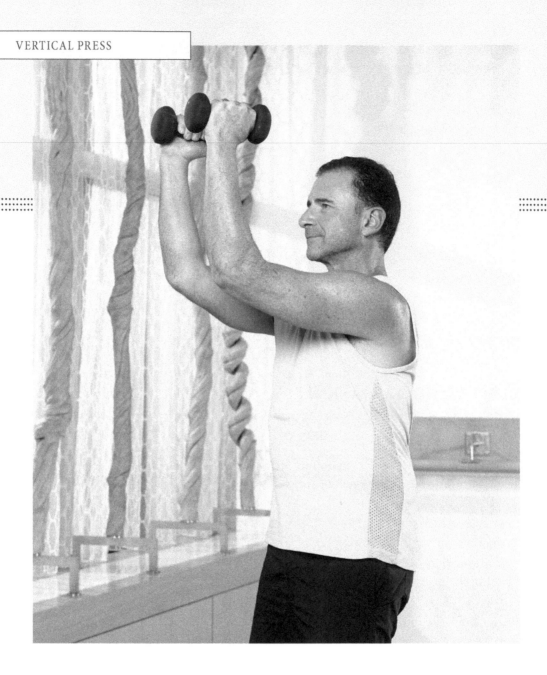

7. On an exhale, lift your elbows a couple of inches (5 cm) above your shoulders, keeping your palms facing each other and your elbows in front of your shoulders.

8. The heads of the weights face forward and your palms face each other.

9. On an inhale, lower your elbows back to shoulder height.

10. Repeat 20 times, lifting your elbows above your shoulders.

>Upper Body<

BICEP CURL, ALTERNATE ARMS

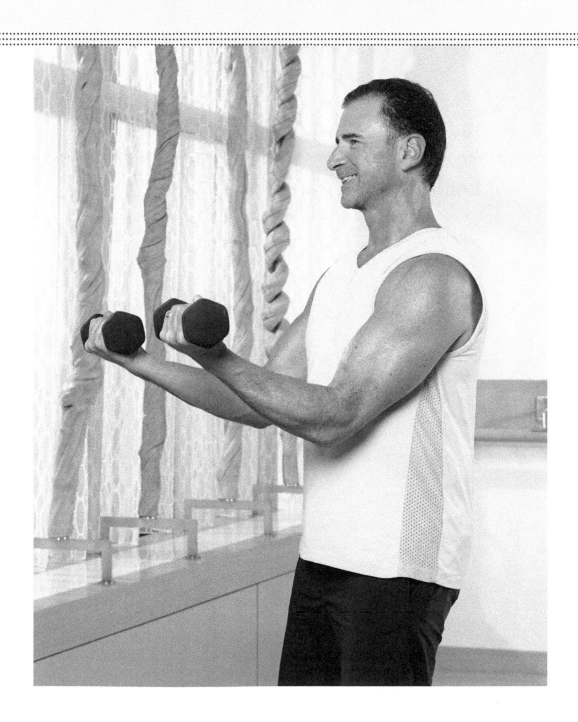

PRIMARY MUSCLES: The biceps brachii, anterior deltoid, brachialis, and bracioradialis are the primary muscles used in this exercise.

STABILIZING MUSCLES: The anterior core/abdominals, thighs and gluteals, rotator cuff, and upper back muscles provide stability.

This exercise uses 2- to 5-pound (1 to 2.5 kg) weights to increase muscular strength in the biceps and creates a muscular balance related to the triceps (back of the upper arms).

SET UP AND BASIC VARIATION

1. Stand with your feet hip-width apart and parallel.

2. Soften your knees over your feet.

3. With 2- to 5-pound (1 to 2.5 kg) hand weights, depending on your level, wrap all your fingers evenly around the stem of the weight.

4. Your ears/shoulders/hips should be stacked on top of each other with even weight distribution over your feet.

5. Maintain a neutral spine and keep your abdominals engaged, feeling the plank energy.

6. Lift your elbows slightly forward from your body in a 90-degree angle below shoulder height and a couple of inches (5 cm) wider than your shoulders.

7. Keep your hands above your elbows, your wrists flat, and your palms facing your shoulders.

WATCH OUT FOR
- *Elbows pressing against hips*

FIX IT
- *Create space to free the shoulder area by taking your elbows away from your hips.*

WATCH OUT FOR
- *Back arching and rocking*

FIX IT
- *Pull in your abdominals and drop your tailbone.*

WATCH OUT FOR
- *Shoulders rising*

FIX IT
- *Settle down your shoulders and use a lighter weight or no weights.*

WATCH OUT FOR
- *Poor posture*

FIX IT
- *Keep your ear/shoulder/hip stacked over each other and your feet parallel to each other, hip-width apart.*

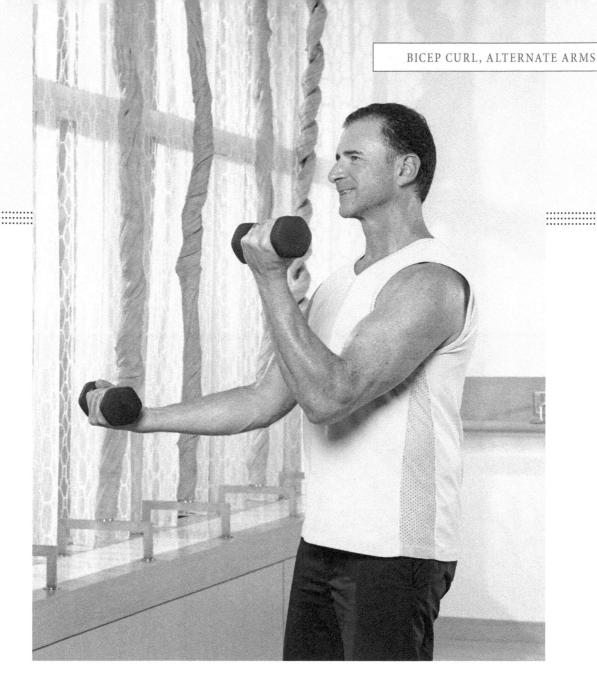

8. Alternately bring the weight/hand toward your shoulder and then to an extended arm position without locking your elbows.

9. Do 30 repetitions, alternating right (counting 1) and left (counting 2).

10. Maintain even breathing; just inhale and exhale normally as you alternate arms.

BICEP CURL, DOUBLE ARMS

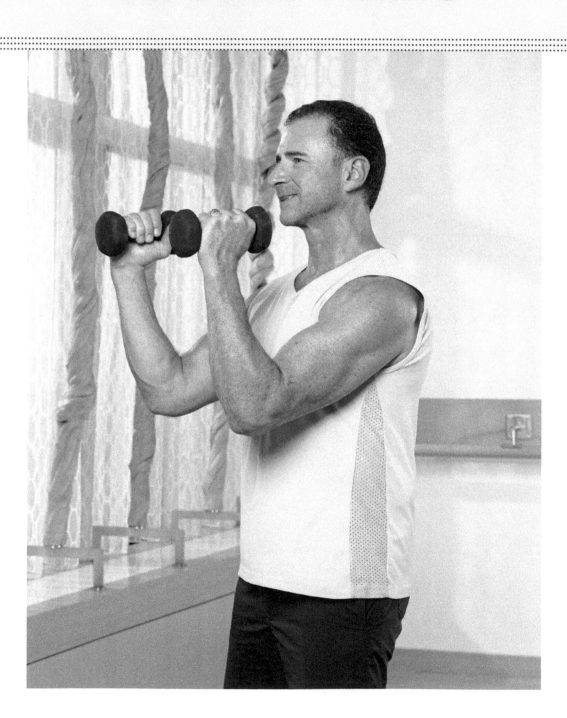

PRIMARY MUSCLES: The biceps brachii, anterior deltoid, brachialis, and bracioradialis are the primary muscles used in this exercise.

STABILIZING MUSCLES: The anterior core/abdominals, thighs and gluteals, rotator cuff, and upper back muscles provide stability.

This exercise uses 2- to 5-pound (1 to 2.5 kg) hand weights to increase muscular strength in the biceps and creates a muscular balance related to the triceps (back of the upper arms). Also, this variation engages more deltoids to strengthen the rotator cuff muscular group.

SET UP AND BASIC VARIATION

1. Stand with feet hip-width apart and parallel.

2. Soften your knees over your feet.

3. With 2- to 5-pound (1 to 2.5 kg) hand weights, depending on your level, wrap all your fingers evenly around the stem of the weight.

4. Keep your ears/shoulders/hips stacked on top of each other with even weight distribution over your feet.

5. Keep a neutral spine and your abdominals engaged, feeling the plank energy.

6. Lift your elbows slightly forward from your body in a 90-degree angle at shoulder height and in front of your shoulders.

7. Keep your hands above your elbows, your wrists flat, and your palms facing your shoulders.

(Continued on next page.)

WATCH OUT FOR
- *Elbows pressing against hips*

FIX IT
- *Create space to free the shoulder area by taking your elbows away from your hips.*

WATCH OUT FOR
- *Back arching and rocking*

FIX IT
- *Pull in your abdominals and drop your tailbone.*

WATCH OUT FOR
- *Shoulders rising*

FIX IT
- *Settle down your shoulders and use a lighter weight or no weights.*

WATCH OUT FOR
- *Poor posture*

FIX IT
- *Keep your ear/shoulder/hip stacked over each other and your feet parallel to each other, hip-width apart.*

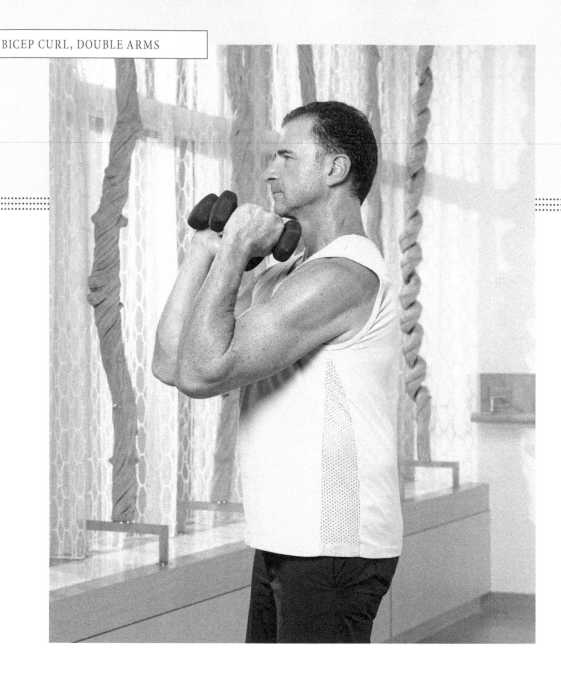

8. On an inhale, bend both elbows and bring the weights/hands toward your shoulders (about 8 to 10 inches [20.5 to 25.5 cm] away from the shoulders). On an exhale, extend/straighten both arms without locking your elbows.

9. Do 30 repetitions of bending and straightening your arms.

TRICEP KICKBACKS

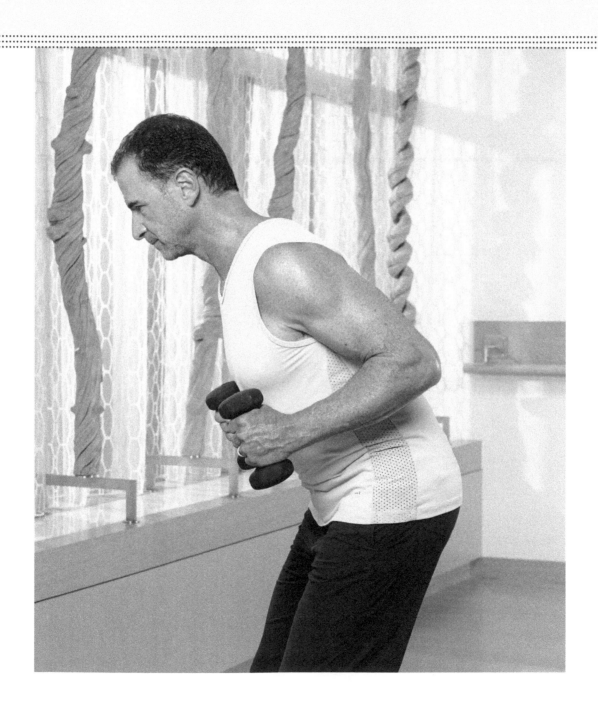

PRIMARY MUSCLES: The triceps and biceps are the primary muscles used in this exercise.

STABILIZING MUSCLES: The erector spinae, anterior and posterior core, thighs, and gluteals provide stability.

One of the most popular areas to tone is the back of the upper arms—the triceps. This exercise, which uses 2- to 5-pound (1 to 2.5 kg) hand weights, also helps to correct slouched posture that may occur from hunching over computers and mobile devices. It's an overall efficient upper-body strengthener. Let's get those triceps toned and flab-free!

SET UP AND BASIC VARIATION

1. Place your feet hip-width apart parallel to each other.
2. With 2- to 5-pound (1 to 2.5 kg) hand weights, depending on your level, wrap all your fingers evenly around the stem of the weight.
3. Hinge forward from your hips with your arms and weights under your shoulder, your palms facing toward each other, and your tailbone dropped.
4. Soften your knees.
5. Tuck under from your waist down and lengthen your spine from your waist up, keeping your middle and upper back in a flat position. Keep your ears in line with your shoulders and your shoulders down.
6. Pull in your abdominals to protect your lower back.
7. Lift both arms straight with your hands above your hips, your arms parallel to the floor, and your palms facing each other.
8. Keeping from elbow to shoulder parallel to the floor, bend your elbows and curl your fists to your shoulders. Keep your arms as close to your body as possible.

WATCH OUT FOR
- *Knees locked, back arched*

FIX IT
- *Soften your knees and pull in and tuck them under to protect your lower back.*

WATCH OUT FOR
- *Arms falling out of position and getting too low at hip level or below hip level*

FIX IT
- *Keep your elbows pressing against your rib cage; use a lighter weight if necessary.*

WATCH OUT FOR
- *Wrist twists*

FIX IT
- *Hold the weights with all your fingers and a light grip. Start with your hand hanging under your shoulder, establish a light grip, and then lift the weight into the correct position using the back of your arm (triceps).*

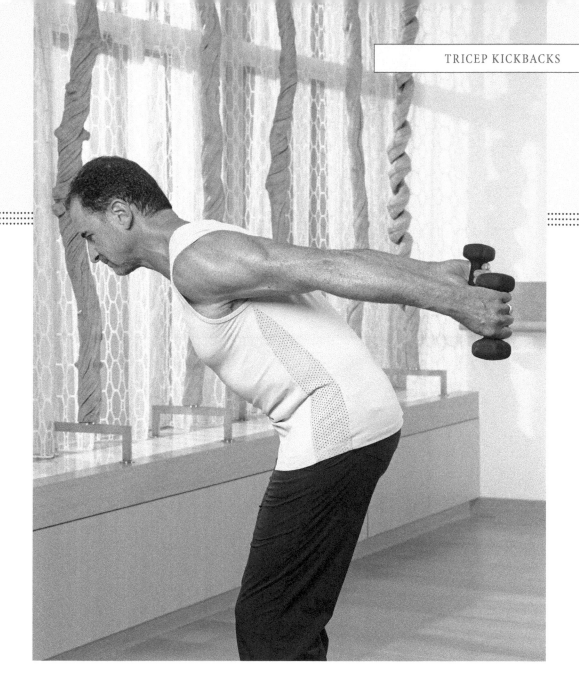

9. Extend both arms from your elbow down to straight arms
   with your palms facing each other.

10. Keep your extended arms parallel to floor and as close to your
    body as possible.

11. Repeat the bend and extension of your arms 10 times.

DOUBLE ARM TRICEPS

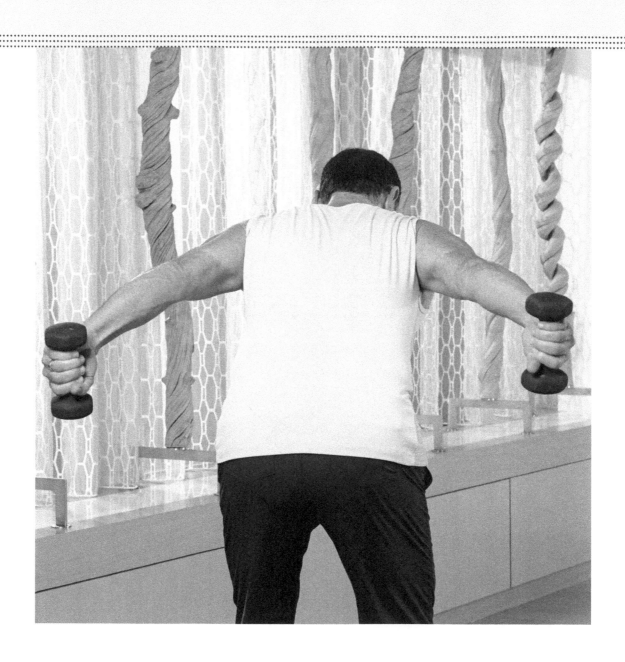

PRIMARY MUSCLES: The triceps, posterior deltoid, and teres major/minor are the primary muscles used in this exercise.

STABILIZING MUSCLES: The erector spinae, anterior and posterior core, thighs, and gluteals provide stability.

Here is some more tricep work to help keep the back of the arms toned. This exercise uses 2- to 5-pound (1 to 2.5 kg) hand weights. Remember that the triceps are a small muscular group, so they are more of a challenge to feel and reshape than bigger muscular groups. We recommend that you do both tricep weight exercises together to thoroughly target them.

SET UP AND BASIC VARIATION

1. Place your feet hip-width apart and parallel to each other.
2. With 2- to 5-pound (1 to 2.5 kg) hand weights, depending on your level, wrap all your fingers evenly around the stem of the weight.
3. Hinge forward from your hips with your arms and weights under your shoulder, your palms facing each other, and your tailbone dropped.
4. Soften your knees.
5. Tuck under from your waist down and lengthen your spine from your waist up, keeping your middle and upper back in a flat position. Keep your ears in line with your shoulders and your shoulders down. Pull in your abdominals to protect your lower back.
6. Lift both arms straight with your hands above your hips and your arms parallel to the floor, and your palms facing each other. Repeat 20 times.

WATCH OUT FOR
- *Knees locked, back arched*

FIX IT
- *Soften your knees and pull in your abdominals to protect your lower back.*

WATCH OUT FOR
- *Arms falling out of position and getting too low at hip level or below hip level*

FIX IT
- *Keep your elbows pressing against your rib cage; use a lighter weight if necessary.*

WATCH OUT FOR
- *Wrists twisting*

FIX IT
- *Hold the weights with all your fingers and a light grip. Start with your hand hanging under your shoulder, establish a light grip, and then lift the weight into the correct position using the back of your arm (triceps).*

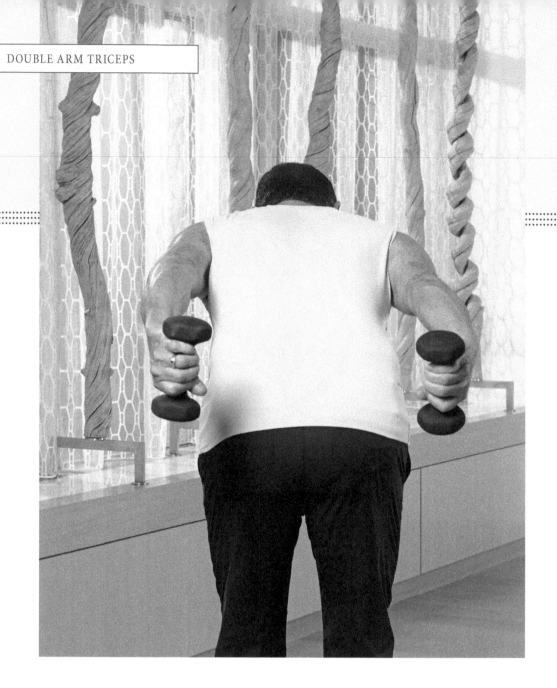

NEXT LEVEL

1. Perform the Set Up for the Basic Variation.

2. Press your upper inner arms against your rib cage while maintaining the height of your arms.

3. Try to avoid any rebound effect; the accent is on the "in" of the movement.

4. Press in your arms to side of your body 20 times.

RHOMBOID ROW

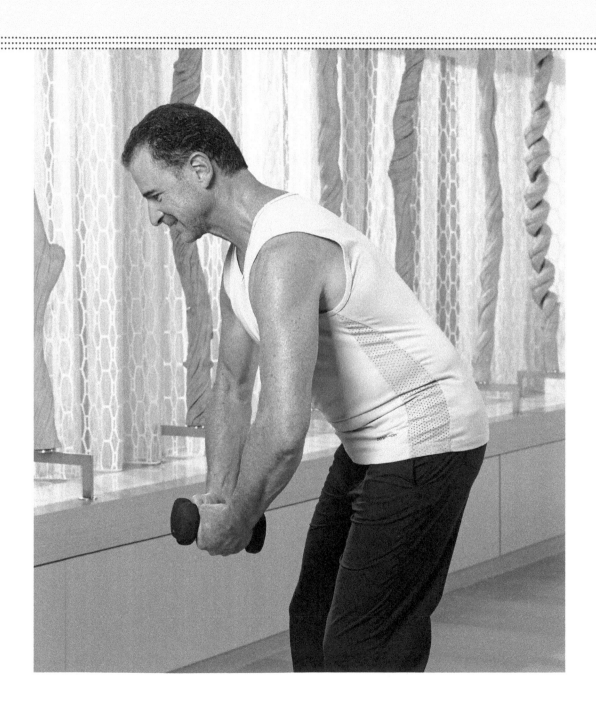

PRIMARY MUSCLES: The rhomboids, trapezius, paraspinal, and the latisimus dorsi; are the primary muscles used in this exercise.

STABILIZING MUSCLES: The anterior core (abdominals) provides stability.

This exercise, which uses 2- to 5-pound (1 to 2.5 kg) hand weights, increases strength and muscle tone between the shoulder blades, which also helps to balance forward-rounded shoulders and tight pectoral muscles. The rhomboid row also helps to improve posture.

SET UP AND BASIC VARIATION

1. Stand with your feet hip-width apart and parallel to each other.
2. With 2- to 5-pound (1 to 2.5 kg) hand weights, depending on your level, wrap all your fingers evenly around the stem of the weight.
3. Keep your knees soft.
4. Keep your abdominals in.
5. Hinge forward from your hips with your arms and weights under your shoulder, your palms facing each other, and your tailbone dropped.
6. Tuck under from your waist down and lengthen your spine from your waist up, keeping your middle and upper back in a flat position. Keep your ears in line with your shoulders and your shoulders down.
7. Bend your elbows to a 90-degree angle with your palms facing toward your sternum (breast bone), about a foot (30.5 cm) away, with your knuckles touching. Your elbows should be below your shoulders.

WATCH OUT FOR
- *Back arching*

FIX IT
- *Pull your abdominals in, and drop your tailbone to a neutral spine.*

WATCH OUT FOR
- *Elbows dropping below shoulders*

FIX IT
- *Switch to a lighter weight.*

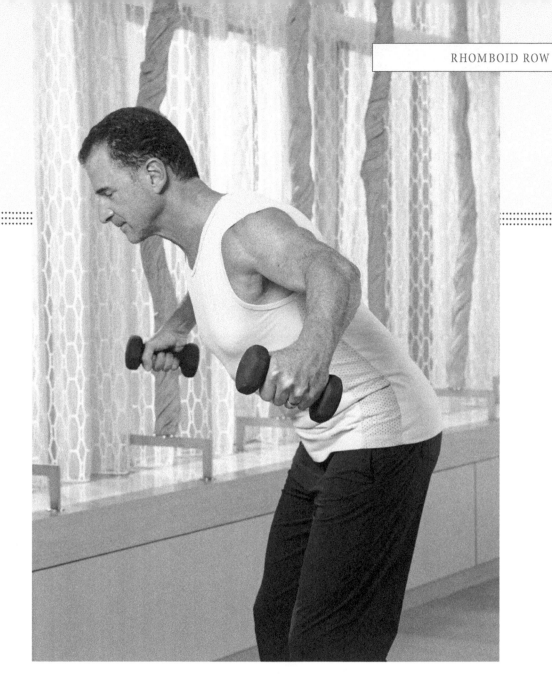

8. With bent elbows, pull the weights apart to above shoulder height, contracting the shoulder blades toward the midline of your body.

9. Exhale as you lift your elbows and inhale as you lower them.

10. Lift and lower your elbows 10 times.

11. Hold the lift and pulse up your elbows 20 times.

TURNED OUT V THIGH

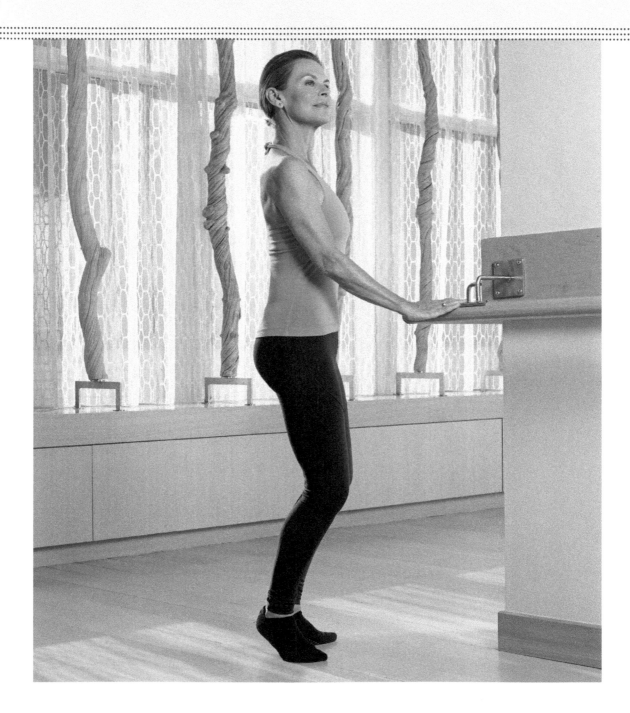

PRIMARY MUSCLES: The quadriceps, abductors, adductors, gastrocnemius, and hamstrings are the primary muscles used in this exercise.

STABILIZING MUSCLES: The abdominals and shoulder girdle provide stability.

Turned Out V Thigh strengthens and elongates the quadriceps group, developing long, lean thighs and calves, helps to stabilize the knee joint, increases muscle density in the quadriceps (not bulk) for optimal caloric usage, and will shed inches. Overall, this exercise decreases total body fat percentage and increases muscle density. The basic variation is good to rehab any knee issues.

SET UP AND BASIC VARIATION

1. Face the barre at arm's length away, your hands placed lightly on the barre at shoulder width apart.

2. Place your heels together and your toes apart in a narrow 45-degree V position. Align your shoulders over your hips and your ears over your shoulders. Your hips, knees, and feet should be stacked on top of each other with any turnout initiating from your hips.

3. Bend your knees about 5 to 6 inches (13 to 15 cm). Raise your heels 2 to 3 inches (5 to 7.5 cm) off the floor, and press your heels together. Soften the elbow(s) of the arm(s) holding the barre.

4. Keep a neutral spine and your abdominals pulled in.

5. Hold for 30 seconds.

6. Return to a standing position.

7. Repeat the pose 3 times.

WATCH OUT FOR
- *Too much turn out*

FIX IT
- *Bring your feet into a smaller 45-degree V position before you begin the movement.*

WATCH OUT FOR
- *Body bouncing at bottom of movement*

FIX IT
- *Slow your movement on the way down and up from the seat to your heels. Keep an even tempo up and down.*

WATCH OUT FOR
- *Lower back tucks under, arches too much, or leans forward toward barre with shoulders up*

FIX IT
- *Bring your shoulders back over your hips while leveling your shoulders. Pull your abdominals in and stay in a neutral spine.*

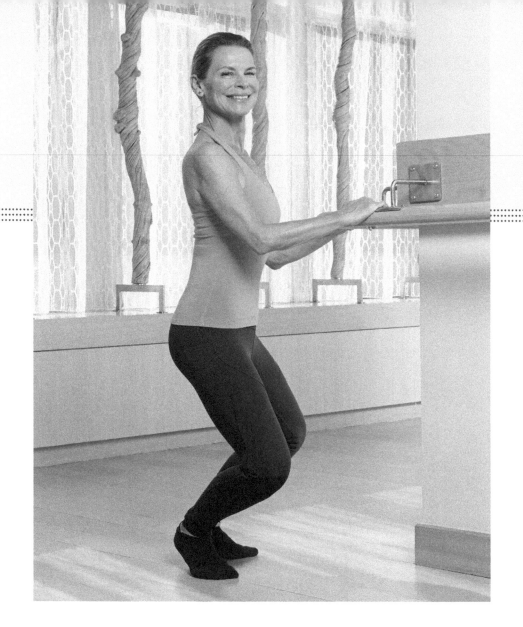

NEXT LEVEL (HALFWAY HOLD OF FULL RANGE)

1. Perform the Set Up and Basic Variation. Bend your knees deeper to feel more thigh engagement.

2. Lower 6 inches (15 cm).

3. For a single count each, lower 2 to 3 inches (5 to 7.5 cm) in position for 20 reps.

4. Perform 20 pulses.

5. Hold the position at the halfway point so that your thighs are in a challenging position.

6. Tuck and release your pelvis 4 times, holding a neutral spine.

7. Balance and hold for 4 counts.

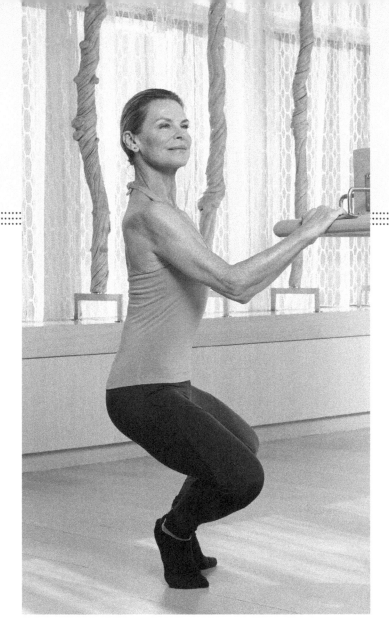

> **NOTE**
>
> A **pelvic tuck** is a posterior tilting of the pelvis from a neutral spine, and the action will lengthen your lower back and will feel like you are lengthening your tailbone away from the crown of your head. The abdominals will pull in and up as the tailbone drops down and under, which in combination creates a pelvic tuck.

ADVANCED (FULL RANGE)

1. Begin from the Halfway Hold position. Because this is more advanced, it should be done facing the barre with both hands on the barre.

2. For a single count each, lower 2 to 3 inches (5 to 7.5 cm) in position for 20 reps.

3. Lower the full range of movement toward your heels (the lowest point is always a few inches [5 to 7.5 cm] above your heels) for 10 reps.

4. Lower to the halfway hold position.

5. Perform 20 pulses.

6. Hold the position at the halfway point so that your thighs are in a challenging position.

7. Tuck and release your pelvis 4 times, holding a neutral spine.

8. Balance and hold for 4 counts, keeping your knees bent and your body in the challenging position of halfway down.

PARALLEL THIGH

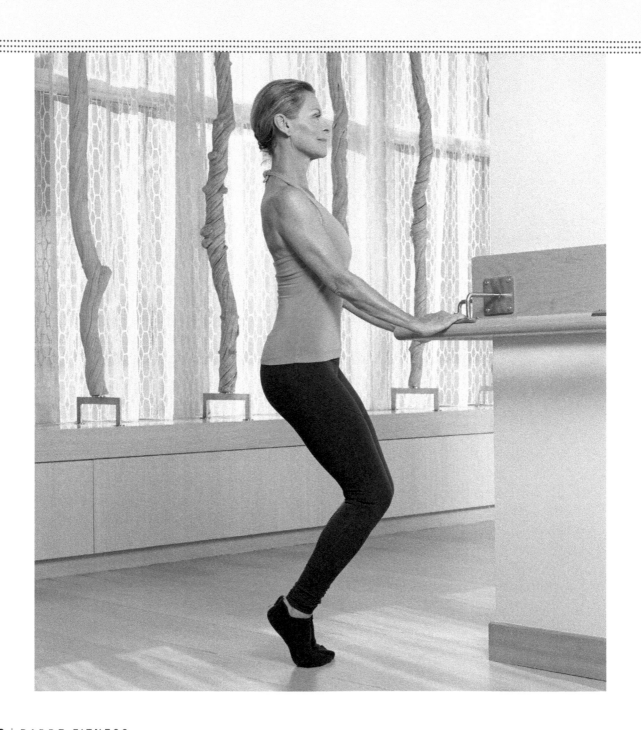

PRIMARY MUSCLES: The quadriceps, adductors, abductors, hamstrings, gluteals, and gastrocnemius are the primary muscles used in this exercise.

STABILIZING MUSCLES: The anterior core (abdominals), forearms, and feet muscles provide stability.

Similar to the Turned Out V Thigh exercise, this exercise strengthens and elongates the entire quadriceps group, developing long, lean thighs and calves. Orthopedically, parallel thigh work helps to stabilize the knee joint. All quadriceps exercises help to increase muscular density in one of the largest muscular groups in the body, the thighs. This then increases the body's capacity for caloric output, decreasing the total body fat percentage and increasing muscle density. An added benefit to this parallel thigh variation is an increased use of the adductors (inner thighs) and abductors (outer thighs).

SET UP AND BASIC VARIATION

1. Facing the barre, step an arm's length away with your feet together.

2. Place your hands lightly on the barre about shoulder-width apart.

3. Keep your ears over your shoulders, your shoulders over your hips, and your knees over your feet.

4. Raise your heels all the way up to the balls of your feet.

5. Bend your knees about 12 inches (30.5 cm), keeping your thighs above knee level.

6. Draw and press both your knees and inner thighs together.

7. Pull your abdominals in and keep a neutral spine.

8. Move your body down and up a couple of inches (5 cm), always keeping your thighs/knees above hip level, along with your tailbone over your heels.

9. Repeat 20 times.

WATCH OUT FOR
• *Knees apart*

FIX IT
• *Press your inner thighs and knees together.*

WATCH OUT FOR
• *Heels too low*

FIX IT
• *Be sure to lift your heels as high as possible with the balls of your feet and all your toes on the floor to stabilize.*

WATCH OUT FOR
• *Shoulders roll forward and back arches*

FIX IT
• *Open and press your shoulders down and back. This helps get your ears over your shoulders and your shoulders over your hips. Keep your eye focus straight ahead. Emphasize pulling your abdominals in to support your back.*

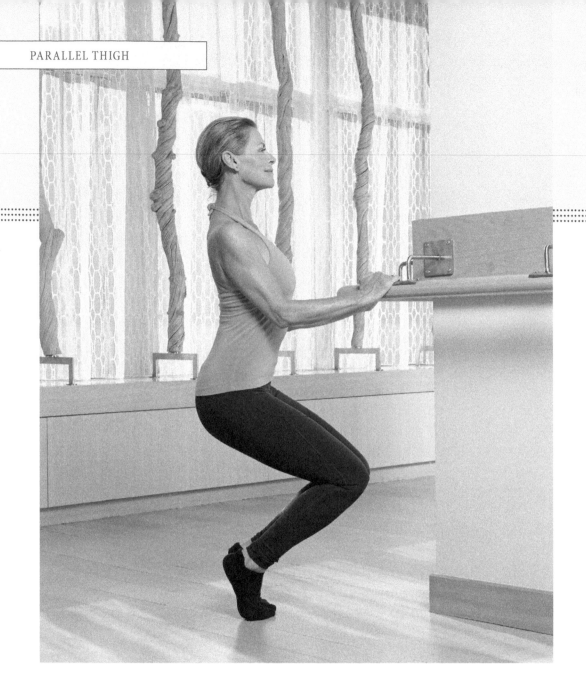

NEXT LEVEL

1. Perform the Set Up and Basic Variation.

2. Bring your hips to knee level and then above knee level 10 times.

3. Hold the last lowering, with your hips at knee level, for 10 seconds.

SINGLE LEG THIGH STRENGTHENERS

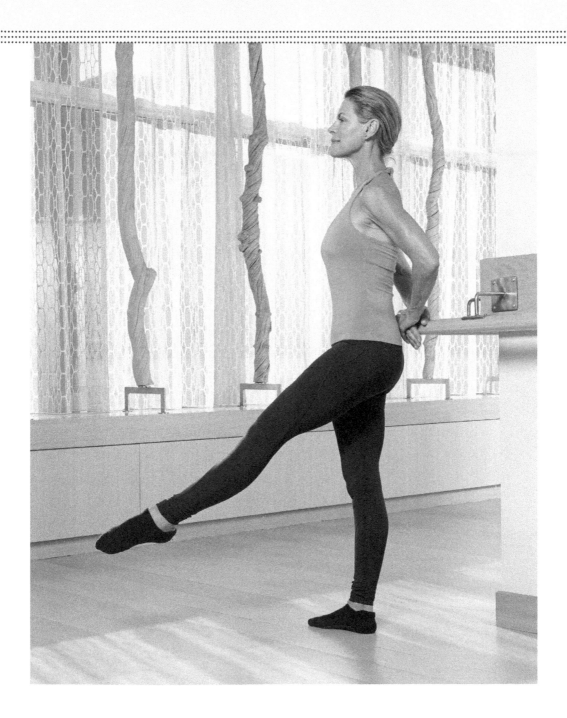

PRIMARY MUSCLES: The quadriceps, gluteals, thigh abductors (outer thighs) and adductors (inner thighs), and gastrocnemius are the primary muscles used in this exercise.

STABILIZING MUSCLES: The anterior core (abdominals) and erector spinae muscles provide stability.

The Single Leg Thigh Strengthener gives you the same benefits as the Turned Out V Thigh exercise along with adding hamstring flexibility. It adds muscular strengthening to the gluteal group and improves balance. Envision yourself with a true dancer's long, lean legs!

SET UP AND BASIC VARIATION

1. Stand about an inch (2.5 cm) away from the barre with your back to the barre.

2. Place your feet in a small turned-out 45-degree V position with your heels together and your toes facing away from each other. Be sure that the turnout of your legs initiates from your hips.

3. Your hips, knees, and feet should align on top of each other.

4. Place your hands behind you on the barre.

5. Keep your elbows bent.

6. Your shoulders remain level and down. Your ears should be over your shoulders, and your shoulders over your hips. Your eye focus should be straight ahead.

7. Pull your abdominals in and maintain a neutral spine.

8. Extend your left leg forward in front of your hip with a pointed, stretched foot, keeping your left leg very straight with your toes on the floor.

9. Keep supporting your standing leg very straight without locking your knee.

WATCH OUT FOR
• *Leaning back with torso*

FIX IT
• *Pull your abdominals up and in.*

WATCH OUT FOR
• *Shoulders rising or uneven*

FIX IT
• *Press your upper back muscles down and together. Keep your ears over your shoulders and your eye gaze forward.*

WATCH OUT FOR
• *Lifted leg bends*

FIX IT
• *Lower your leg a little and stretch your hamstrings.*

WATCH OUT FOR
• *Standing leg bends*

FIX IT
• *Lift and engage your gluteal muscles along with lengthening your hamstrings on your standing leg.*

WATCH OUT FOR
• *Losing balance*

FIX IT
• *Lift your abdominals up and in. Lean slightly forward to your lifted leg.*

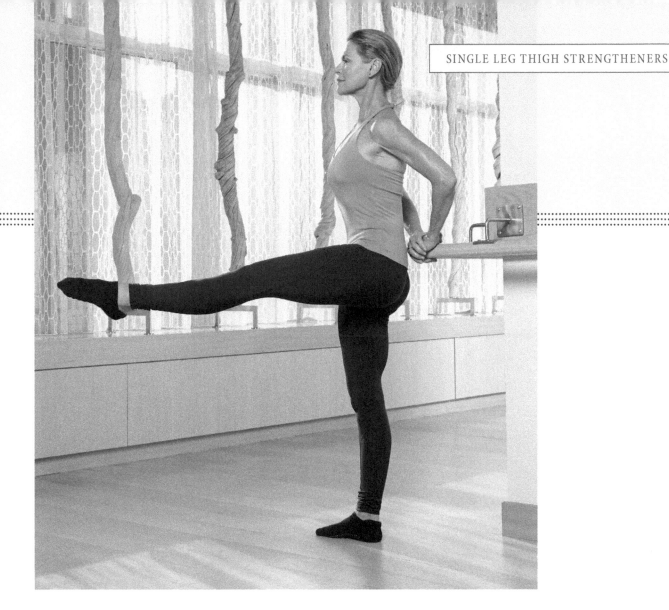

10. Lift both your hands off the barre for a moment to assess correct weight distribution and then lightly touch the barre again.

11. Raise your foot/leg about 1 to 2 feet (30.5 to 61 cm) off the floor.

12. Hold for 10 seconds.

13. Lower your leg to the floor and lift 10 times.

14. Hold the last lift and then lower and lift your leg a couple inches (5 cm) down and up 10 times.

15. Release your left leg and repeat all with your right leg.

NEXT LEVEL

1. Perform the Set Up and Basic Variation.

2. Raise your right foot/leg to hip height.

3. Hold for 10 seconds.

4. Lower your leg to the floor and lift 10 times.

5. Hold the last lift and then lower and lift your leg a couple inches (5 cm) down and up from hip height 10 times.

6. Release your right leg and repeat all with your left leg.

SINGLE LEG LUNGE

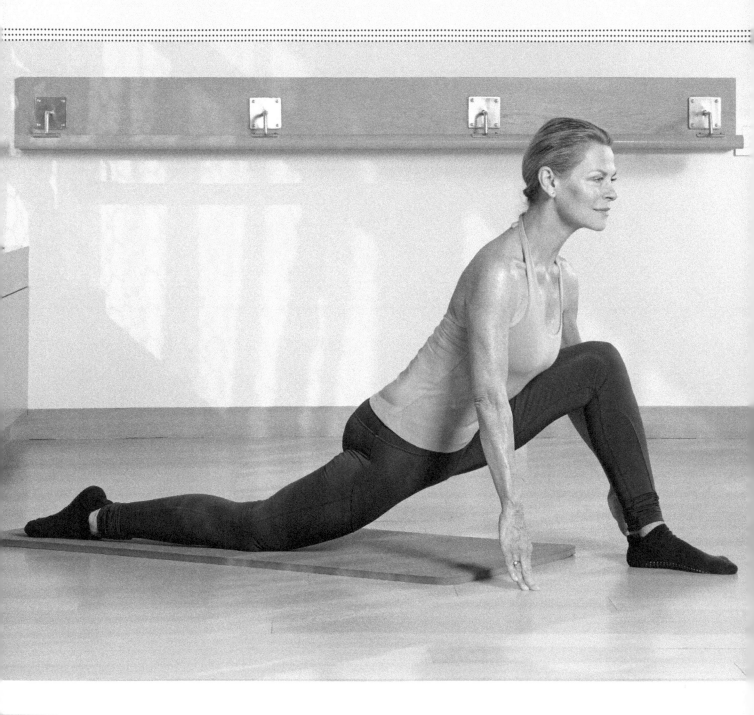

PRIMARY MUSCLES: The thighs and hip flexors are the primary muscles used in this exercise.

STABILIZING MUSCLES: The shoulder muscles pressing down, abdominals, and arm muscles provide stability.

This Single Leg Lunge stretch increases the flexibility of the thighs and hip flexors to help create long, lean functional thigh muscles. This helps to balance the strengthening and shortening of the thigh muscles, allowing you greater range of movement in the legs. Remember to maintain fluid breathing throughout the stretch and exhale when pressing to elongate the muscles.

SET UP AND BASIC VARIATION

1. Your left foot lunges forward with your ankle bone under your knee and your hips facing forward and level.

2. Your legs are hip-width apart.

3. Extend your right leg back behind your body, placing this knee on the floor, with your hips pressing forward to open and stretch your back leg hip flexors and thigh muscles. Shift your body weight forward on a diagonal off your back knee cap and more into the lower thigh right above your knee cap.

4. Your front foot should have its weight distributed evenly through all four corners of your foot.

5. Your back foot should have its weight down the center of your foot.

6. Place your hands on the floor, one to each side of your front foot, with your palms facing each other.

7. Keep your abdominals pulled in and lifted off your front thigh.

8. Hold for 30 seconds and repeat with your right leg forward.

WATCH OUT FOR
- *Front knee bends to outside or inside of body or too far forward*

FIX IT
- *Be sure your front knee is above your ankle bone, along with your knee being in front of your hip. Also make sure your front foot is facing straight forward.*

WATCH OUT FOR
- *Hips misaligned*

FIX IT
- *Turn your back hip down and inward.*

WATCH OUT FOR
- *Straining muscles*

FIX IT
- *Emphasize the exhale as you stretch deeper. Move slowly in and out of the stretch. Place your hands on top of your front thigh instead of the floor.*

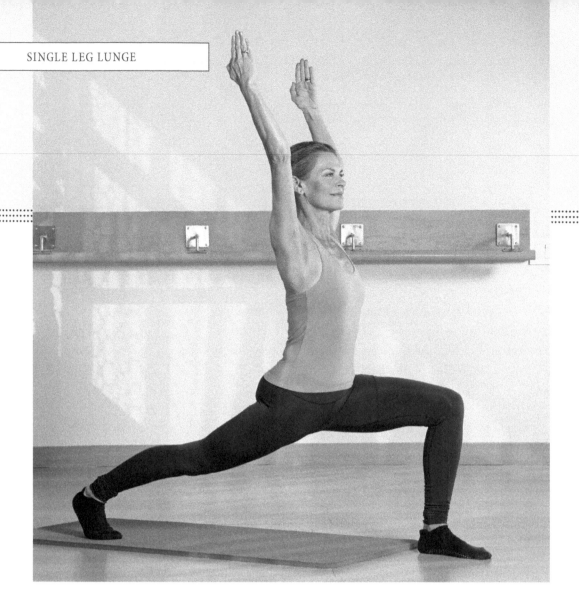

NEXT LEVEL

1. Perform the Set Up and Basic Variation.

2. Move your left leg forward.

3. Keep your right leg back, tuck your toes under, stretch your leg straight, and press through the ball of your foot.

4. Inhale to extend your arms above your shoulders, shoulder-width apart, with your palms facing each other. Press your shoulders down.

5. Your eyes should gaze straight ahead with your chin parallel to the floor.

6. Keep your abdominals in and elongate out of your hips.

7. Bring your upper body weight back over your pelvis to increase the stretch.

8. Avoid overarching your back; instead, think of lifting up and over, creating more space in your lower back and more length in your spine.

9. Hold for 30 seconds and let the exhale take you deeper and more relaxed into the stretch.

10. Repeat with your right leg forward.

HAMSTRING/ CALF STRETCH

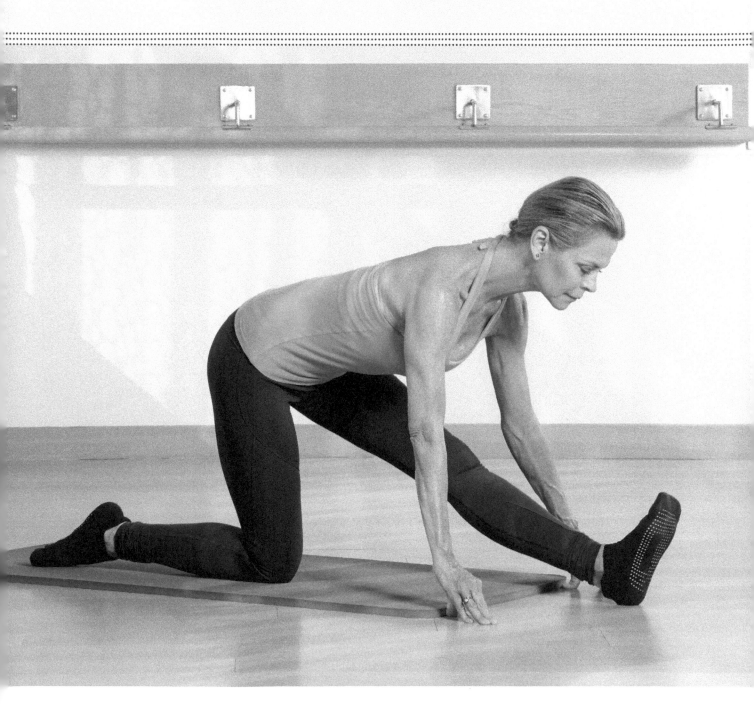

PRIMARY MUSCLES: The hamstring group and gastrocnemius (calf muscles) are the primary muscles used in this exercise.

STABILIZING MUSCLES: The abdominals support the lower back, with the shoulder muscles pressing down to lengthen the spine.

The Hamstring/Calf Stretch helps to increase flexibility in the back of the leg and hamstring area. It also increases the range of movement in the pelvic area, which in turn relieves lower back pain. These muscles tend to be very tight when you spend a lot of time sitting. Look forward to long, lean, functional hamstring muscles with this stretch.

SET UP AND BASIC VARIATION

1. Your right knee, shin, and foot should be on the mat or a padded surface with your left leg straight and extended forward in front of your hip with your foot flexed.

2. Keep your right hip in alignment above your right knee.

3. Your legs should be hip-width apart and your hips facing forward.

4. Lengthen your spine from your tailbone to the crown of your head. Keep your neck in alignment with your spine. Keep your ears over your shoulders.

5. Place the fingertips of both hands on the floor, straddling the front leg, with your arms shoulder-width apart so your shoulders can press down.

6. Exhale and reach your chest toward your front thigh. Hold for 30 seconds.

7. Repeat with the other leg in front.

WATCH OUT FOR
- *Over-stretching*

FIX IT
- *Encourage patience, focus, and breath. Relax your facial muscles.*

WATCH OUT FOR
- *Misalignment*

FIX IT
- *Move slowly into the stretch, keeping your hips level.*

WATCH OUT FOR
- *Top leg bends*

FIX IT
- *Bring your torso up higher and walk your hands closer to your hips. Avoid bringing your leg too far forward.*

WATCH OUT FOR
- *Uneven hips*

FIX IT
- *Square your hips by pulling in your abdominals and leveling your hips.*

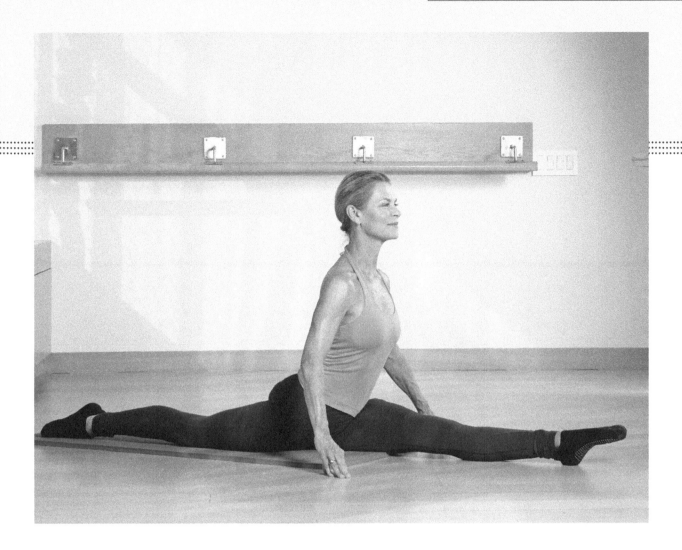

NEXT LEVEL

1. Perform the Set Up and Basic Variation.

2. Slide your left leg forward as far as possible with your hips remaining parallel. Achieve this by pulling your left hip back and leading the movement with your back right hip rotating down and forward.

3. Only go as far forward as you can while keeping your front left leg straight. If it starts to bend, stay higher up.

4. Place your hands or elbows on the floor, one on each side of the front leg.

5. Exhale deeper when you have arrived at your full front leg extension. Hold for 30 seconds.

6. Repeat with other leg in front.

STANDING GLUTEAL

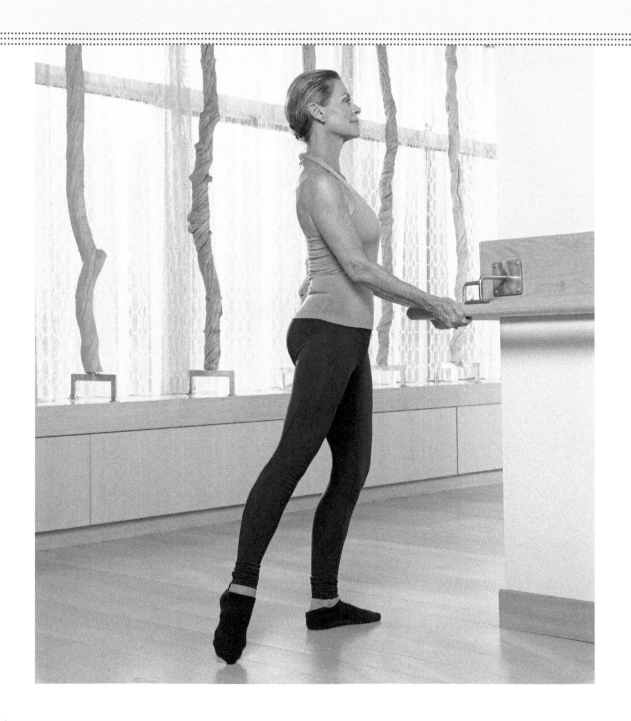

PRIMARY MUSCLES: The gluteals, tensor fascia latte, abductors, gastrocnemius, and soleus are the primary muscles used in this exercise.

STABILIZING MUSCLES: The abdominal wall, gluteals (on standing leg), upper inner thighs, and posterior shoulder girdle provide stability.

This is one of the best classic barre standing gluteal exercises because it not only gives you a high, round, lifted butt, but it is also a weight-bearing exercise that improves bone density. It is also great for reshaping the calf muscles to help give you that true dancer aesthetic—long, lean legs, lifted glutes, and improved posture.

SET UP AND BASIC VARIATION

1. Facing the barre, stand about a forearm's distance away with your feet hip-width apart and parallel and with an underhand grip on the barre. Keep your ears over your shoulders and your shoulders over your hips.

2. Stretch the top of your right toes and foot into the floor, on a five o'clock diagonal line. Soften into both knees, pull your abdominals in, drop your tailbone, and slightly tuck under.

3. Straighten your right leg with your foot pointed and the back of your leg straight.

4. Turn out your right leg only from the hip, keeping it behind your standing leg.

5. Shift your body weight to the inside edge of your standing foot, keeping even weight distribution over your standing foot.

6. Keep your hips square and facing forward as your working leg is turned out from your inner hip joint.

(Continued on next page.)

WATCH OUT FOR
- *Working lower back instead of gluteals*

FIX IT
- *Drop your tailbone and lengthen your lower back more. Pull in your abdominal wall and reduce the range of motion.*

WATCH OUT FOR
- *Locking the standing knee and sitting in the standing hip*

FIX IT
- *Soften your standing knee and keep your body weight on the inside edge of your standing foot.*

WATCH OUT FOR
- *The working leg swings front to back. When this happens, the correct muscles will not engage because the movement needs to be more controlled toward a back-only direction, eliminating the forward swing.*

FIX IT
- *Add a back hold between each movement done with a straight leg and your foot off the floor. The goal is to break the momentum and build a momentary pause into each repetition.*

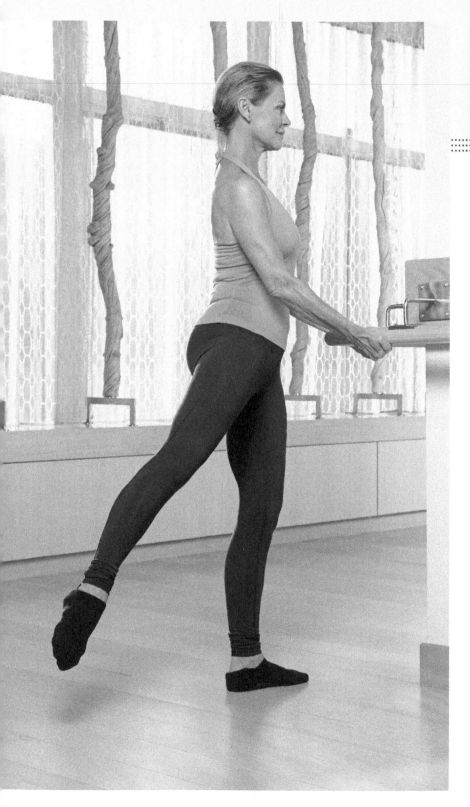

When picturing the alignment of this exercise, visualize a clock. If you are facing 12 o'clock, then directly to your rear is 6 o'clock, your direct right side is 3 o'clock, and your direct left side is 9 o'clock. In order to properly set up this exercise, you will extend your working leg behind your hip on a 5 o'clock angle called a right side diagonal if it's your right leg or to the 7 o'clock angle or left side diagonal if it's your left leg.

7. Lift your right leg off the floor, keeping your foot turned out.

8. Press your leg back and hold 10 times.

9. Press your leg back without a hold and more of a flowing movement 20 times.

10. Lift your leg on a side diagonal with a hold 10 times.

11. Lift your leg on a side diagonal without a hold and more of a flowing movement 20 times.

12. Alternate a press-back and a lift to the side on the diagonal 10 times.

13. Repeat on the other leg.

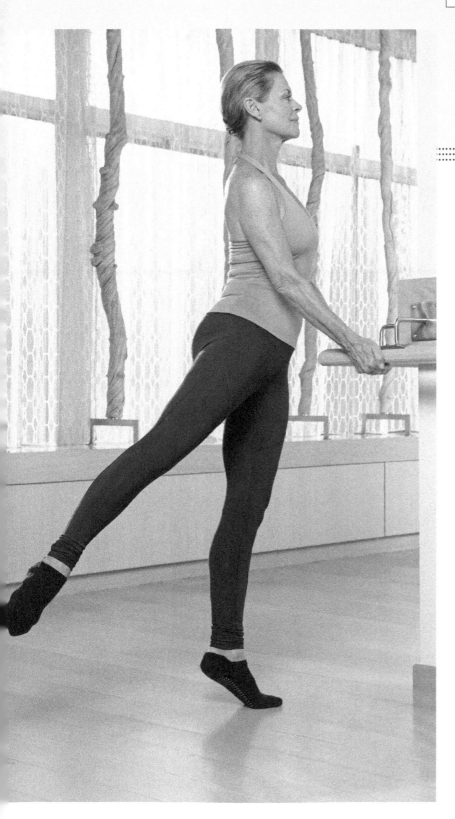

ADVANCED VARIATION

1. Perform the Set Up for the Basic Variation.

2. Raise your standing heel while keeping your standing knee soft. Keep your foot pointed on your working leg. Finish with 10 side diagonal up and hold.

3. Repeat on the other leg.

FIGURE 4

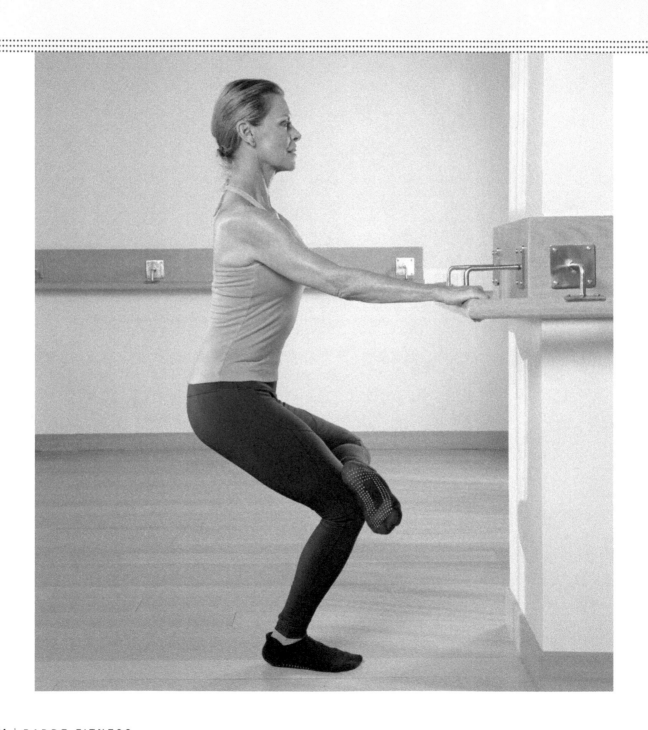

PRIMARY MUSCLES: The gluteals, hip abductors and adductors are the primary muscles used in this exercise.

STABILIZING MUSCLES: The arm muscles, shoulder girdle muscles, and quadriceps provide stability.

The Figure 4 Stretch helps to stretch the gluteals and hip abductors and adductors. This is also a very thorough lower-back stretch, especially if you sit or stand for long periods of time. This exercise, when done regularly, will give you more flexible hips and lower back.

SET UP AND BASIC VARIATION

1. Face into the barre an arm's length away and shoulder-width apart. Your palms should face down on the barre.
2. Keep your legs parallel and hip-width apart.
3. Bend both knees and cross your left ankle over your right lower thigh.
4. Bend deeper into your standing leg to create a deeper opening of your hip area.
5. Allow your left thigh to drop toward the floor.
6. Keep your shoulders down and level and your eye gaze straight ahead.
7. Pull back from the barre with straight arms.
8. Keep your abdominals pulled in.
9. Maintain a flat back that is upright and straight.
10. Exhale deeper once you arrive in the full stretch. Hold for 30 seconds.
11. Repeat with the other leg.

WATCH OUT FOR
- *Standing foot turns out*

FIX IT
- *Position the toes of your standing foot to face directly to the barre.*

WATCH OUT FOR
- *Arms bend too much and shoulders lift*

FIX IT
- *Pull back from the barre more so your arms are fully extended.*

WATCH OUT FOR
- *Lower back arches*

FIX IT
- *Pull in your abdominals and slightly let your pelvis/ tailbone drop to the floor.*

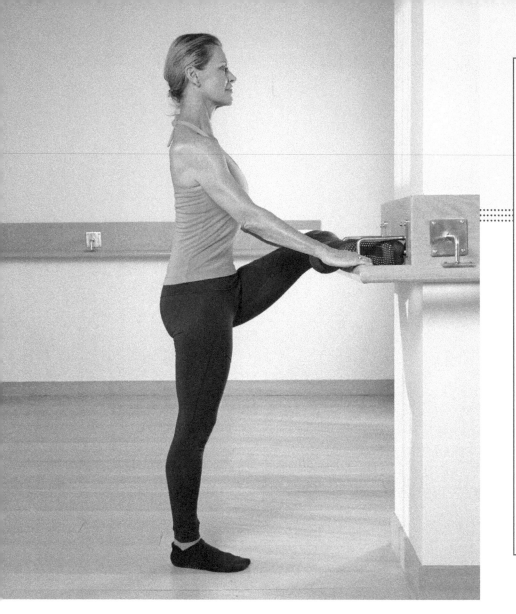

WATCH OUT FOR
• *Standing leg bends*

FIX IT
• *Pull up your standing leg using your quadriceps. Press your heel into the floor.*

WATCH OUT FOR
• *Shoulders rise*

FIX IT
• *Press your shoulders down and engage your upper back muscles.*

WATCH OUT FOR
• *Leg angle is too narrow on barre*

FIX IT
• *Step back from the barre and move your knee in front of your hip.*

NEXT LEVEL

1. Perform the Set Up and Basic Variation.
2. Place your left ankle on the barre with your shin parallel to the barre.
3. Keep your left knee and ankle in a straight line.
4. Your left knee is in front of your left hip at a 90-degree angle.
5. Your shin may or may not touch the barre.
6. Keep your standing leg straight with your hip, knee, and ankle stacked on top of each other. All five toes should be on the floor facing the barre.
7. Keep your back straight and flat with your abdominals pulled in.
8. Keep your eye gaze forward and your shoulders down.
9. Initiate the stretch from your lower back and hips.
10. Exhale deeper into the stretch. Hold for 30 seconds.
11. Repeat with the other leg.

PRETZEL

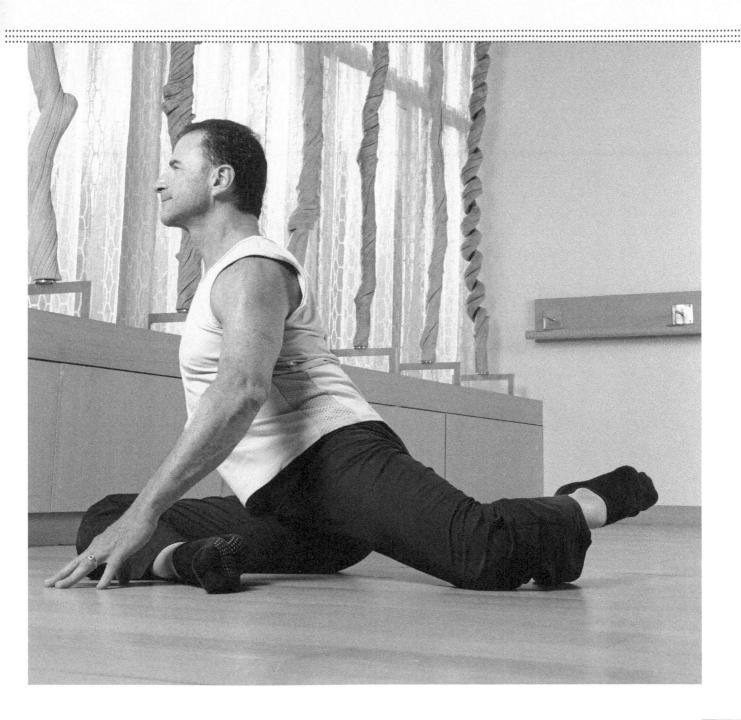

PRIMARY MUSCLES: The gluteus minimus and medius, TFL, vastus lateralis, and quadratus lumborum are the primary muscles used in this exercise.

STABILIZING MUSCLES: The abdominals, latissimus, and rhomboids provide stability.

The Pretzel is a gluteal strengthener as well as a side core stabilizer, which makes it a great exercise for shaping the waist and high glute area. The position will challenge a biker with tight hip flexors in flexibility, as well as challenge the athlete to keep the knee behind the hip while seated in the position. That is the beauty of the pretzel; it is a multi-dimensional exercise capable of a multitude of results.

SET UP AND BASIC VARIATION

1. Sit with your left knee behind your hip and the right knee directly in line with your right hip.

2. Square your breast bone over the center of your front thigh, sitting with your ears over your shoulders and hips. Your abdominals are pulled in with your shoulders pressing down.

3. Rotate your left hip (the working hip) forward so that your left ankle comes off the floor and release.

4. Isolate this movement so that your upper body is still and just your back hip/leg moves.

5. Repeat 10 times.

6. Hold the last repetition for 10 seconds.

7. Repeat this sequence with your right leg.

WATCH OUT FOR
- *Working knee moves in front of hip*

FIX IT
- *Your hip flexors must be stretched open to support the position, which requires your working knee to be behind your hip at all times.*

WATCH OUT FOR
- *Leaning far away from center*

FIX IT
- *Being able to lift the support hand, which is opposite of the working leg at any time, is a good reference for proper pretzel positioning.*

WATCH OUT FOR
- *Ankle of the working leg falls below knee height*

FIX IT
- *The proper pretzel position has the working hip inwardly rotated throughout the exercise. If your ankle falls below your knee, you have lost the position and a reset is needed.*

WATCH OUT FOR
- *Shoulders lifting*

FIX IT
- *Shoulder lifting is one of the first signs that you are straining. Press your shoulders down and back, especially when the exercise is in motion.*

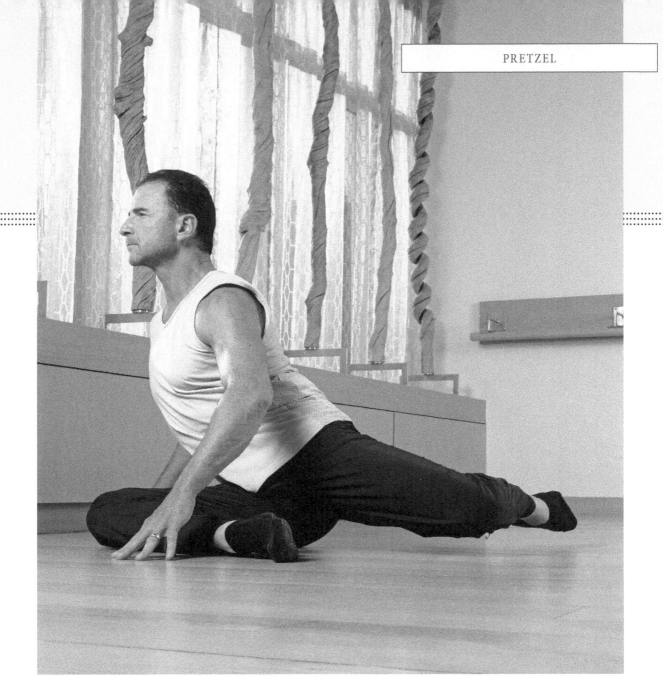

NEXT LEVEL

1. Repeat the Set Up and Basic Variation and then lift and lower your left knee while maintaining the position.

2. Repeat 10 times.

3. Hold the last repetition for 10 seconds.

4. Repeat this sequence with your right leg.

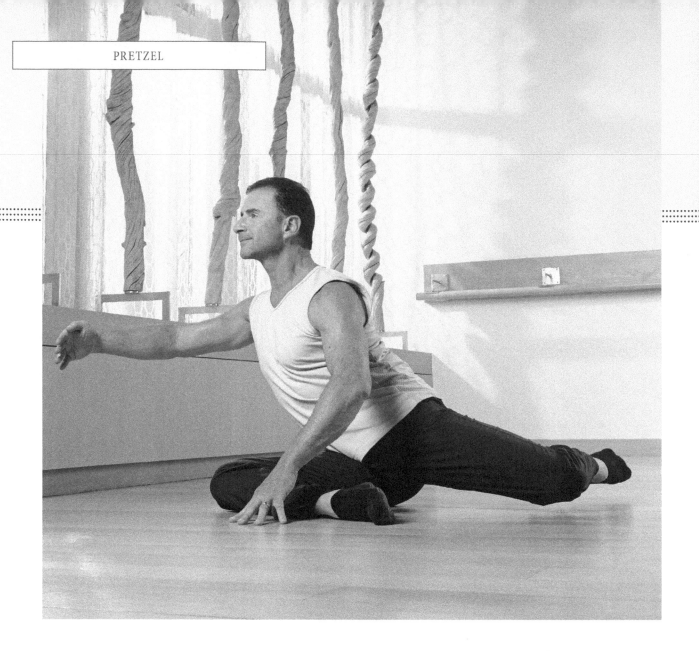

ADVANCED VARIATION

1. Repeat the Set Up and Basic Variation.

2. Repeat the lifting and lowering of your knee.

3. Lift the opposite arm shoulder high while also lifting your knee.

4. Repeat 10 times.

5. Hold the last repetition for 10 seconds.

6. Repeat this sequence with your other leg.

PRETZEL
WITH SEATED TWIST

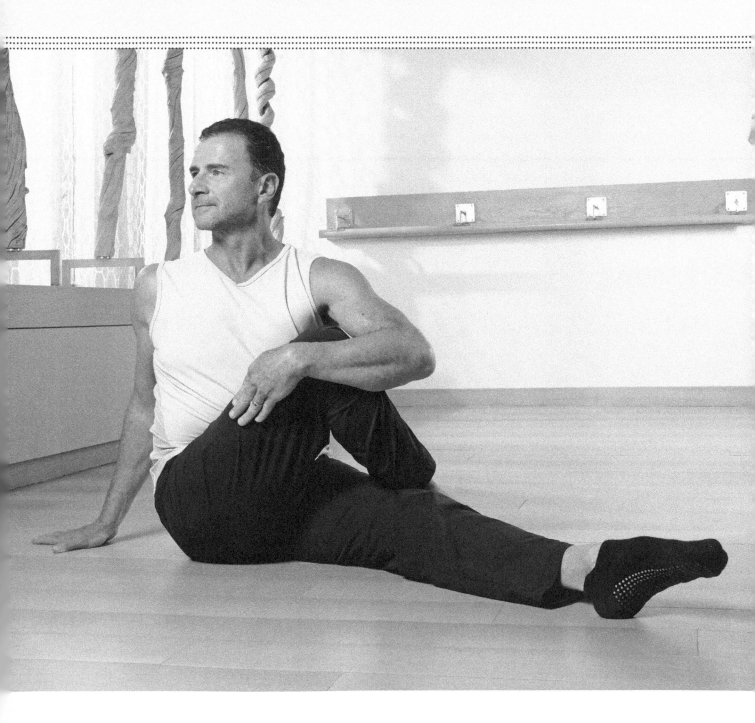

PRIMARY MUSCLES: The gluteus minimus and medius, TFL, vastus lateralis, and quadratus lumborum are the primary muscles used in this exercise.

STABILIZING MUSCLES: The abdominals, latissimus, and rhomboids provide stability.

This position will stretch the muscles used in the Pretzel. The standard Pretzel is a strengthening position. This position is a stretch that complements the standard Pretzel.

SET UP AND BASIC VARIATION

1. Sit on the floor with both legs straight out in front of your hips.
2. Bend your right knee and step that foot across your left thigh.
3. Use your left arm to hug your bent knee toward your chest as your body spirals toward your right (top) leg.
4. Use your back hand against the floor to prop up your posture with your shoulders down and the center of your body lifted.
5. Hold the stretch for 3 deep, slow breaths.
6. Repeat on the other side.

WATCH OUT FOR
- *Hip of the top leg lifts off the floor*

FIX IT
- *Shift your body weight down and toward your top hip. Always keep your bottom leg straight.*

WATCH OUT FOR
- *Back rounds in poor posture*

FIX IT
- *Use your back hand/arm to push down into the floor and lift your spine/back against this action. Pull in your abdominals and open/drop your shoulders.*

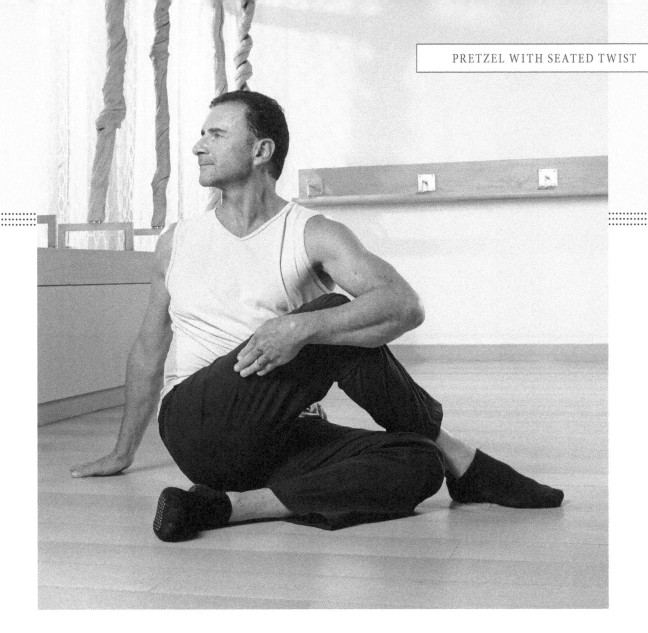

NEXT LEVEL

1. Sit on the floor with both legs straight out in front of your hips.

2. Bend your right knee and step that foot across your left thigh.

3. Use your right arm to hug your bent knee toward your chest as your body spirals toward your right (top) leg.

4. Just before the complete spiral, lean back slightly and bend your left knee.

5. Position the left heel away from your sitz bone, which needs to be grounded into the floor.

6. Use the back of your hand against the floor to prop up your posture with your shoulders down and the center of your body lifted.

7. Hold the stretch for 3 deep breaths.

8. Repeat on the other side.

FLAT BACK

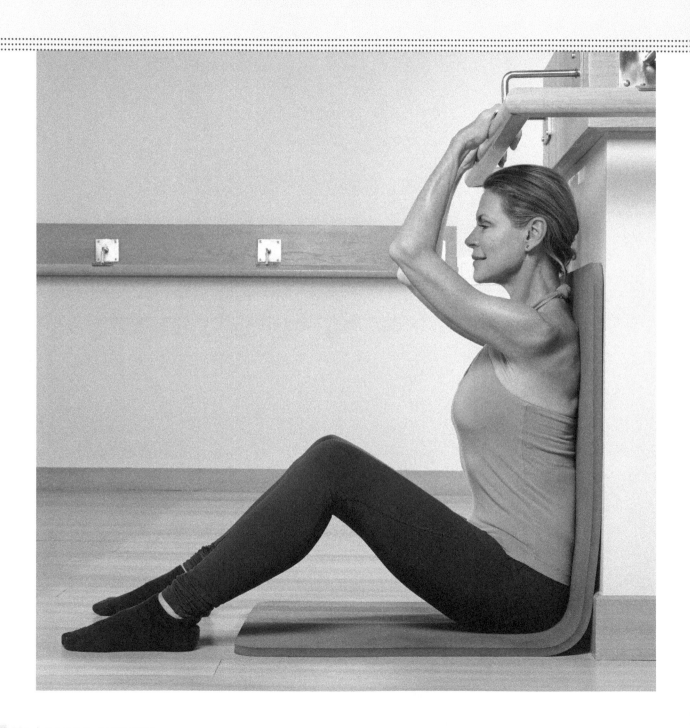

PRIMARY MUSCLES: The abdominals, hip flexors and quadriceps are the primary muscles used in this exercise.

STABILIZING MUSCLES: The abdominals, latissimus, and rhomboids provide stability.

This position will help you build strength in your core muscles. The abdominals must pull in toward the spine in order to engage your core. The exercise will challenge you to hold the abdominals in while your legs are moving under that bracing or pulling in of the abdominal muscles.

SET UP AND BASIC VARIATION

1. Walk your hips into the mat/wall until there is no space behind your lower back. Round up into the seated position with your knees bent, your feet flat, and your legs parallel to each other.

2. Pull down on the barre with both hands facing down and your arms shoulder-width apart.

3. Pull your abdominals in at your center and breathe without releasing the abdominals.

4. Open and close your legs with your feet on the floor. Focus on keeping your abdominals pulled in while your legs are moving under the bracing or pulling in ofthe abdominals.

5. Repeat 20 times, maintaining a flat back that is straight upright.

WATCH OUT FOR
- *Abdominals are pushing out instead of pulling in*

FIX IT
- *Sit in stillness and hold your abdominals in while breathing. Breathe without releasing the abdominals. Keep your abdominals pulled in while you are doing the exercise.*

WATCH OUT FOR
- *Shoulders lifting up*

FIX IT
- *Reduce the intensity of the exercise and press your shoulders down while you are doing the exercise.*

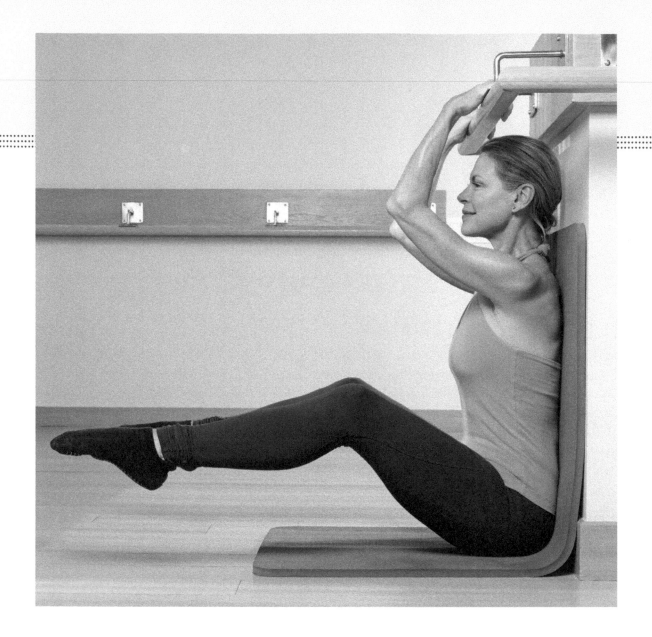

NEXT LEVEL

1. Perform the Set Up and Basic Variation.

2. Lift your feet off the floor while doing the open/close leg movements and keep your abdominals pulled in while your legs are in motion.

3. Repeat 20 times.

FLAT BACK WITH STRAIGHT LEGS

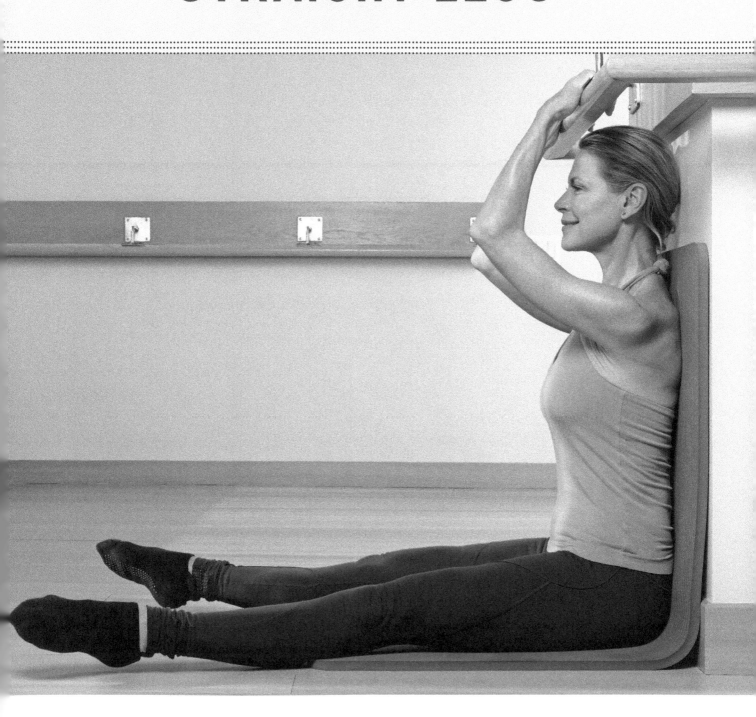

PRIMARY MUSCLES: The abdominals, hip flexors, and quadriceps are the primary muscles used in this exercise.

STABILIZING MUSCLES: The abdominals, latissimus, and rhomboids provide stability.

This position will help you build strength in your core muscles. The abdominals must pull in toward the spine in order to engage your core. The exercise will challenge you to hold your abdominals in while your legs are moving under that bracing or pulling in of the abdominal muscles.

SET UP AND BASIC VARIATION

1. Walk your hips into the mat/wall until there is no space behind your lower back. Round up into the seated position with your legs straight and turned out and your feet pointed and on the floor.

2. Pull down on the barre with both hands facing down and your arms shoulder-width apart.

3. Pull your abdominals in at your center and breathe without releasing the abdominals.

4. Open and close your legs with your feet on the floor with a focus on keeping your abdominals pulled in while your legs are moving under the bracing or pulling in of the abdominals.

5. Repeat 20 times.

WATCH OUT FOR
- *Abdominals pushing out instead of pulling in*

FIX IT
- *Sit in stillness and hold your abdominals in while breathing. Breathe without releasing the abdominals. Keep your abdominals pulled in while you are doing the exercise.*

WATCH OUT FOR
- *Shoulders lifting up during the exercise*

FIX IT
- *Reduce the intensity of the exercise and press your shoulders down while you are doing the exercise.*

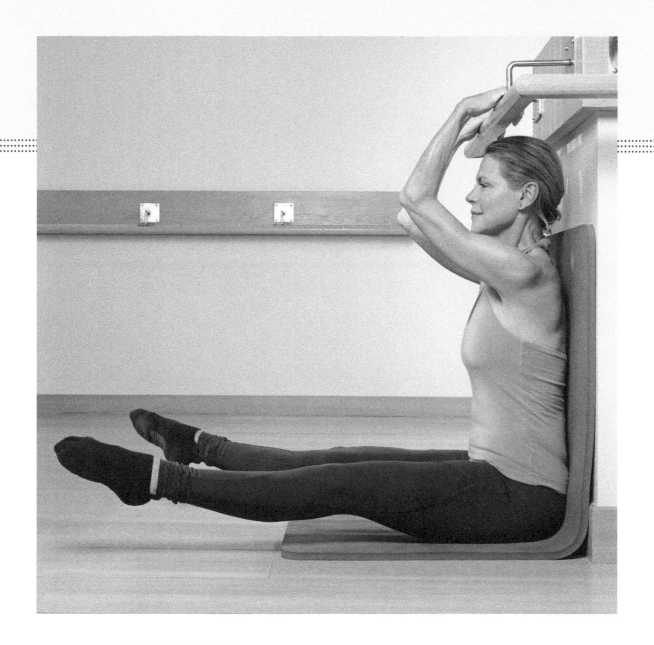

NEXT LEVEL

1. Perform the Set Up and Basic Variation.
2. Lift your feet off of the floor while doing the open/close leg movements and keep your abdominals pulled in while your legs are in motion.
3. Repeat 20 times.

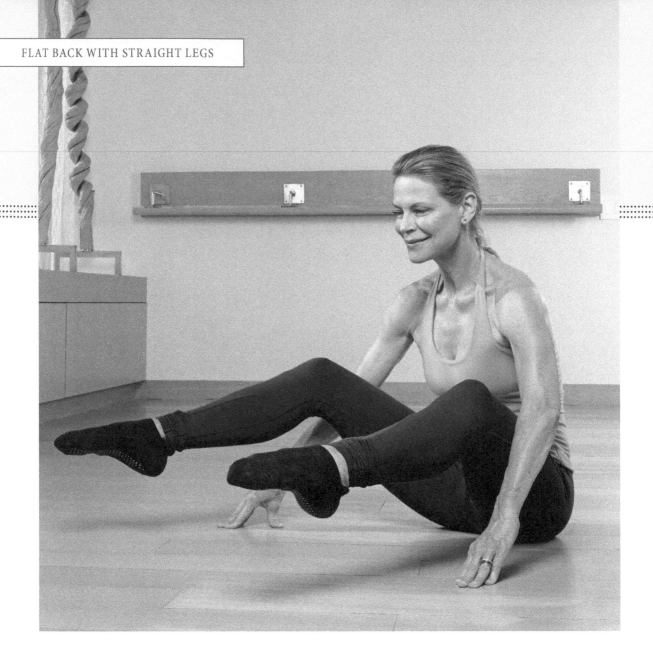

BARRE-LESS VARIATION

1. Sit away from the wall with your knees bent, your feet flat, your upper body leaning forward, and your arms on the outside of your legs with weighted fingertips pressing into the floor.

2. Pull your abdominal muscles in and keep them pulled in while you are doing the open and close exercise with your feet on the floor.

3. Repeat 20 times.

4. The next level is to lift your feet off the floor while doing the open and close exercise (see page 106).

ROUND BACK

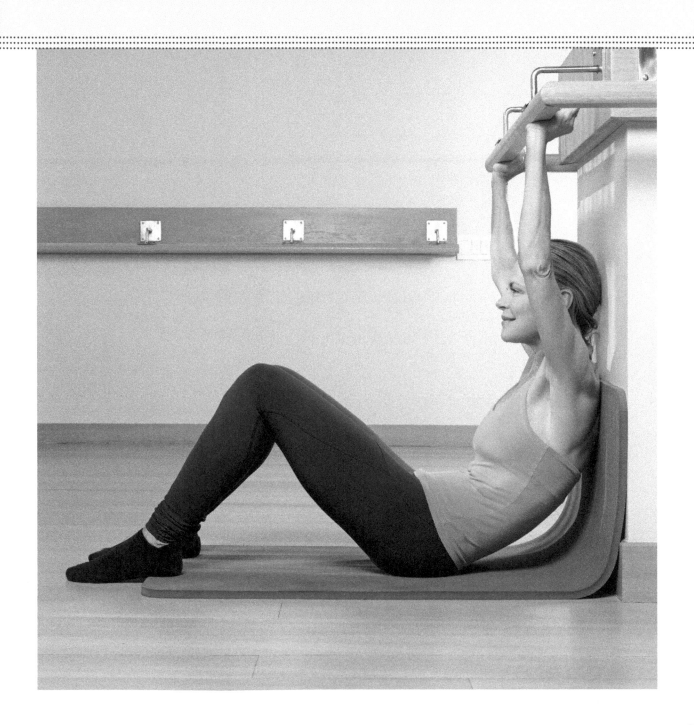

PRIMARY MUSCLES: The abdominals, hip flexors, and quadriceps are strengthening, and the back body muscles are stretching.

STABILIZING MUSCLES: The abdominals, latissimus, and rhomboids provide stability.

This position will help you to build strength in your core muscles. The abdominals must pull in toward the spine in order to engage your core. The added benefit to doing the Round Back position is the back flexibility component. Your posterior muscles are stretching while your anterior muscles are strengthening, thus creating a perfectly balanced position.

SET UP AND BASIC VARIATION

1. Sit under the barre with your shoulder blades on the wall and your spine in a slightly rounded position. The back of your waist should be off the mat.
2. The hands should press up under the barre about shoulder-width apart with a slight bend in your elbow.
3. Your knees are bent, and your feet are flat on the floor.
4. Pull your abdominal muscles in and breathe without releasing your abdominals. Your arms press up and your shoulders drop while your abdominals pull in, and the combination of these forces creates the position.

WATCH OUT FOR
- *Abdominals pushing out instead of pulling in*

FIX IT
- *Sit in stillness and hold your abdominals in while breathing. Breathe without the abdominals releasing; they stay pulled in the entire time.*

WATCH OUT FOR
- *Shoulders lifting up*

FIX IT
- *Reduce the intensity of the exercise and press your shoulders down.*

WATCH OUT FOR
- *Hands pulling down instead of pushing up*

FIX IT
- *Open your palms and press up under the barre while pressing your shoulders down.*

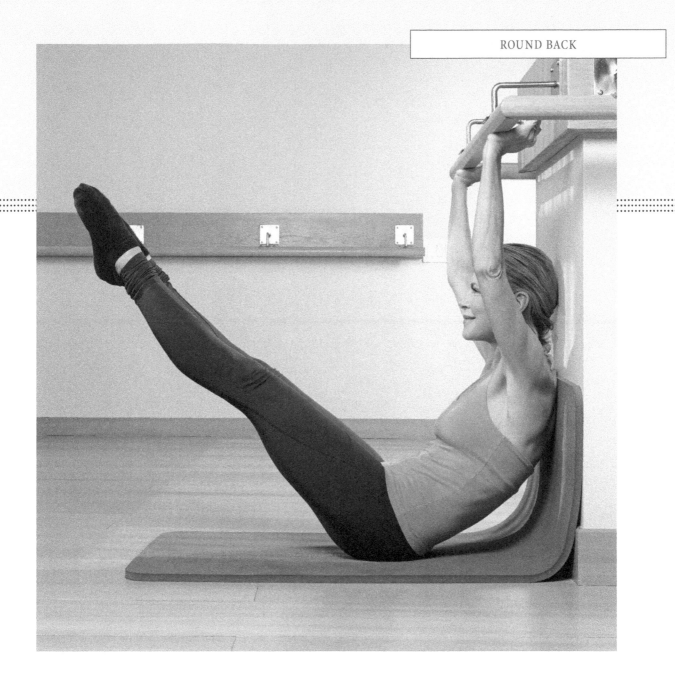

NEXT LEVEL

1. Establish the position as described in the Basic Variation, and then extend one leg to a 45-degree angle very slowly, pulling your abdominals in deeper as your leg extends.

2. Repeat on the other leg.

3. Alternate your legs 5 times to each side.

4. Do the same movement with both legs at the same time.

5. Repeat 5 times.

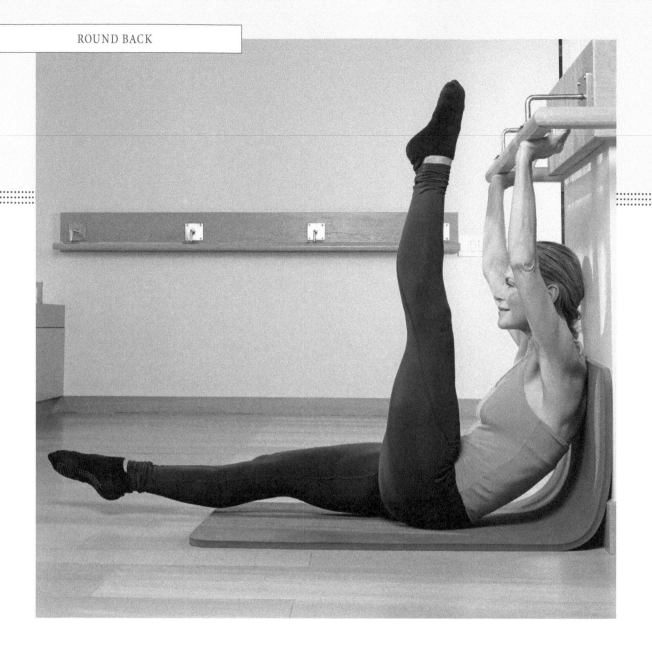

ADVANCED VARIATION 1

1. Establish the position as described in the Basic Variation.

2. Extend one leg along the floor and the other leg above the hip, creating a 90 degree angle with your legs.

3. Hold your top leg with one hand while pressing up under the barre with your other hand. Lift your bottom leg a few inches (5 to 7.5 cm) off the floor.

4. Pull your abdominal muscles in and hold the position for 10 seconds.

5. Repeat on the other leg.

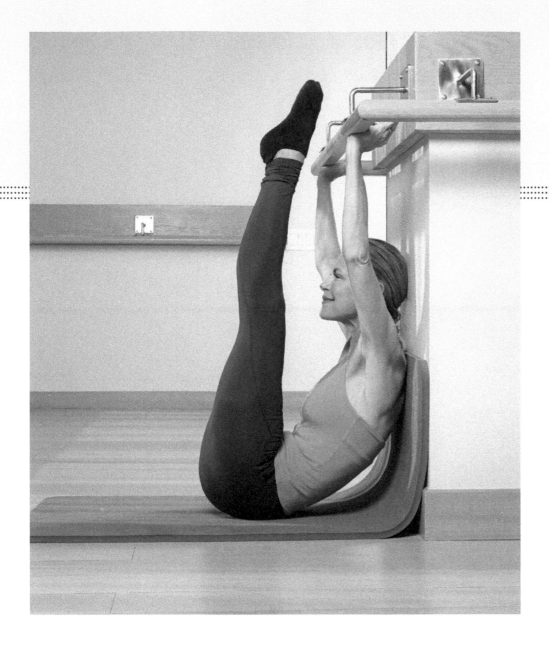

ADVANCED VARIATION 2

1. Establish the position as described in the Basic Variation.

2. Extend both legs up above your hips with your knees straight and your feet pointed.

3. Press both palms up under the barre while pulling your abdominals in toward your spine.

4. Hold the position for 10 seconds.

5. Hug your knees into your chest.

>Abdominals and Core<
CURL

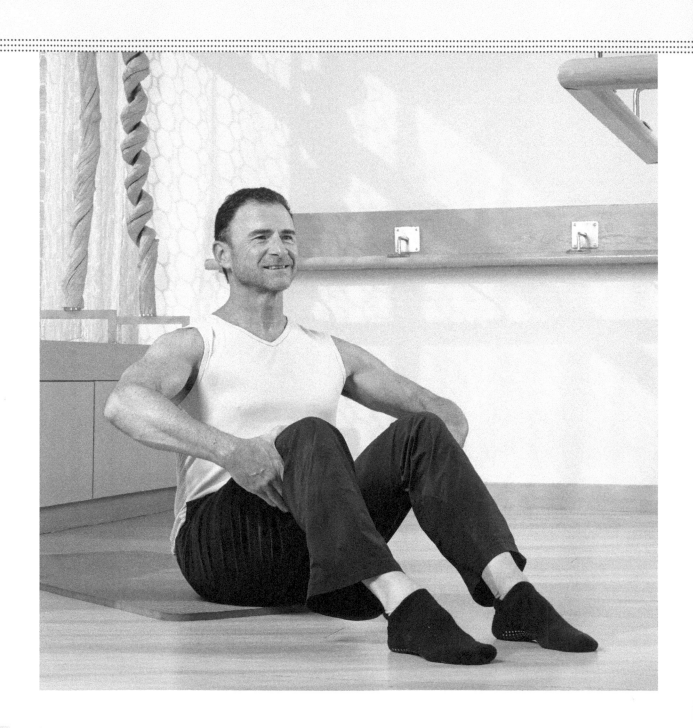

PRIMARY MUSCLES: The abdominals are strengthening, and the back body muscles are stretching.

STABILIZING MUSCLES: The abdominals pull in, and the latissimus and rhomboids (shoulders) press down.

This position will help you build strength in your core muscles. The abdominals must pull in toward the spine in order to engage your core. The added benefit to doing the Curl position, similar to Round Back, is the stretching of the back muscles while the abdominal muscles strengthen.

SET UP AND BASIC VARIATION (OPTION 1)

1. Sit upright with your knees bent, your feet flat, and your hands holding your outer thighs. Your elbows are bent wide to the sides, and your shoulders press down. Your ears are lined up over your shoulders with the bottom of your chin parallel to the floor.
2. Roll down to your waist from a seated upright position while maintaining proper form.
3. Repeat rolling down and up 5 times.
4. Hold on the waist after 5 times for 10 seconds.

WATCH OUT FOR
- *Abdominals pushing out instead of pulling in*

FIX IT
- *Sit in stillness and hold your abdominals in while breathing. Breathe without the abdominals releasing; they stay pulled in the entire time.*

WATCH OUT FOR
- *Shoulders lifting up*

FIX IT
- *Reduce the intensity of the exercise and press your shoulders down.*

WATCH OUT FOR
- *Neck compensates for lack of abdominal use*

FIX IT
- *Work a little higher up in the position in the beginning and keep your head properly aligned over your shoulders.*

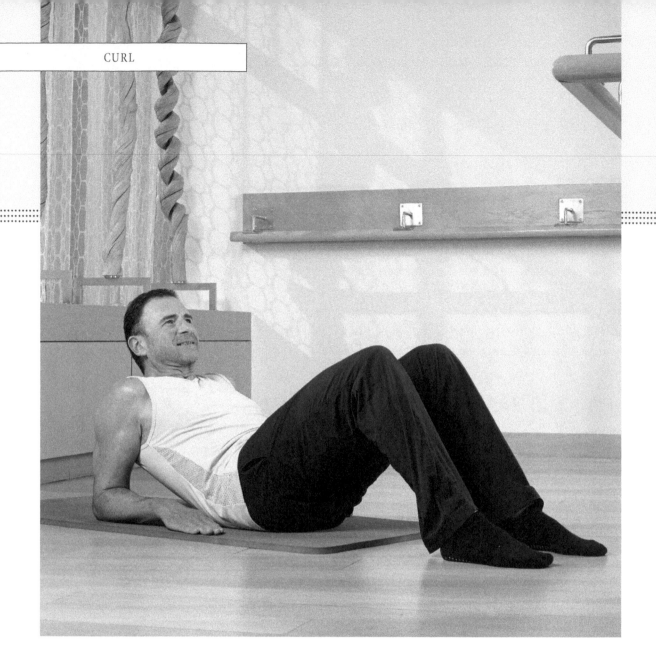

SET UP AND BASIC VARIATION (OPTION 2)

1. Sit with your knees bent, your feet flat, and your elbows resting on the floor, slightly behind your shoulders with your palms down.

2. Pull your abdominal muscles in toward your spine and tuck your pelvis under in order to press your lower back down into the mat.

3. Hold this position and practice breathing without moving the abdominals for 10 seconds.

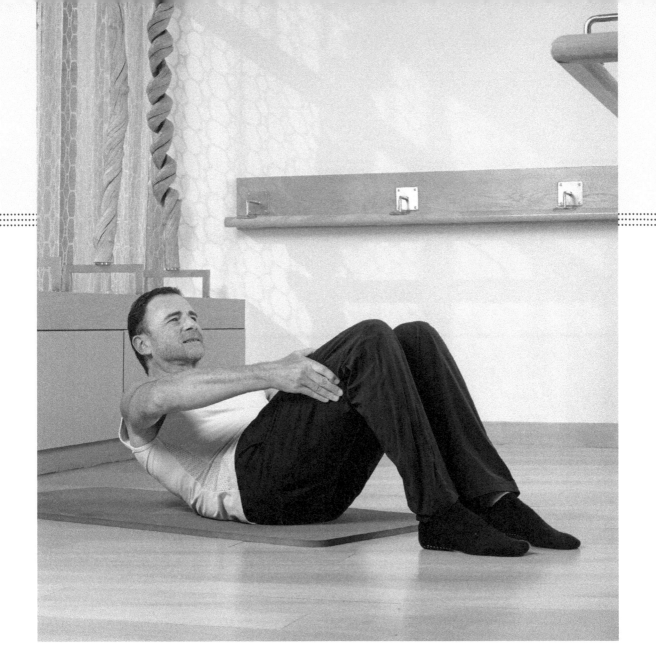

STARTING POSITION

1. Use the Basic Variation (option 1) to initiate the Set Up position.

2. Hold on to your outer thighs while pressing your lower back down into the floor.

3. When holding your outer thighs, your elbows are high and wide, your shoulders are down and back, your ears are over your shoulders, and the bottom of your chin is parallel to the floor.

4. Hold the position for 10 seconds and then rest and repeat 5 times.

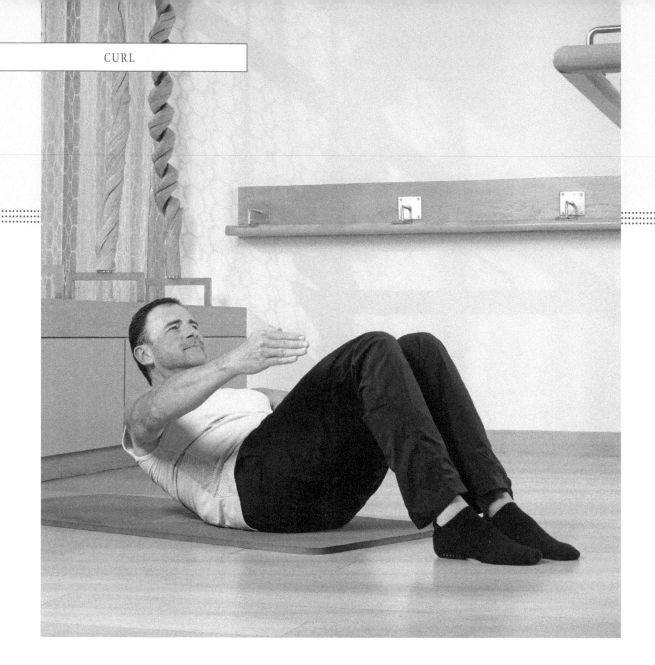

NEXT LEVEL

1. Use the Basic Variation (option 1) to initiate the Set Up position.

2. Establish and hold your Starting Position. Once you can hold the position for 10 seconds, try to take one hand off your leg.

3. Take both hands off your leg and hold the position for 10 seconds.

4. Rest and repeat 5 times.

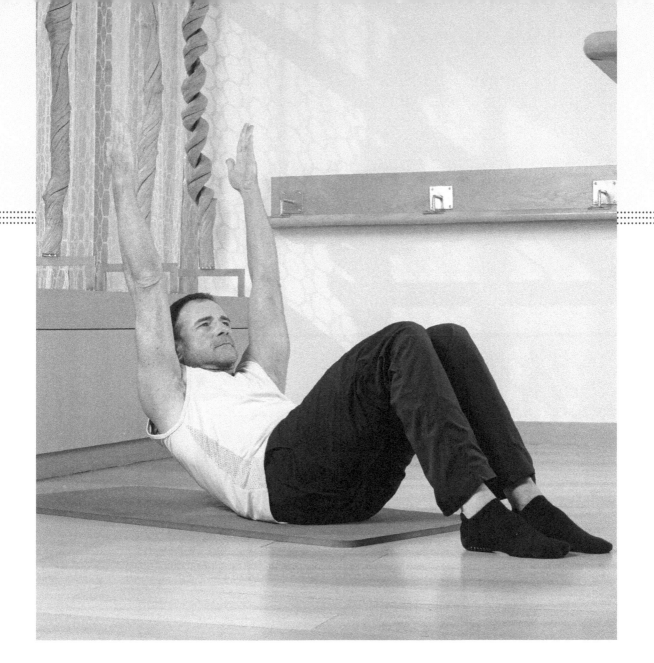

ADVANCED VARIATION

1. Once you can hold the Starting Position and Next Level, proceed to the more advanced level and raise both arms.

2. Rest and repeat 5 times.

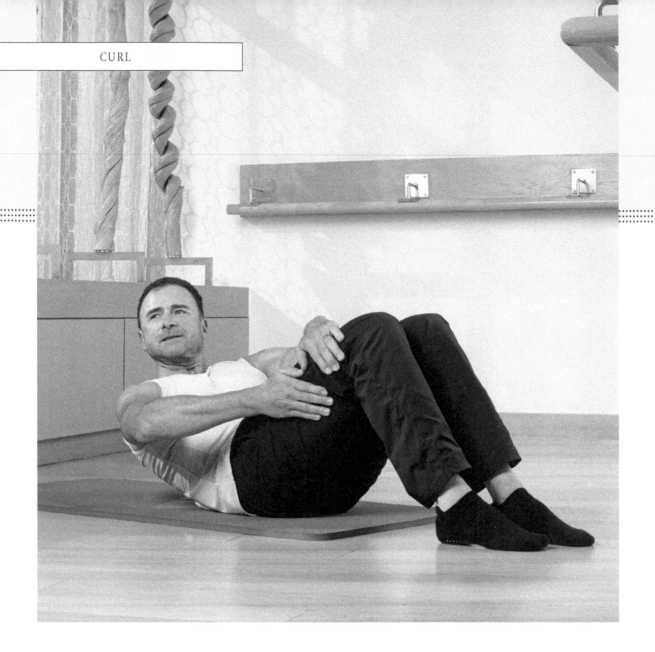

OBLIQUES WITH BENT KNEES

1. Hold the Starting Position.
2. Bring your left hand to your right outer thigh as you twist your upper body to the left.
3. Hold on with both hands and stay in the position without falling back or coming up.
4. Hold the position for 10 seconds.
5. Rest and repeat on the other side.

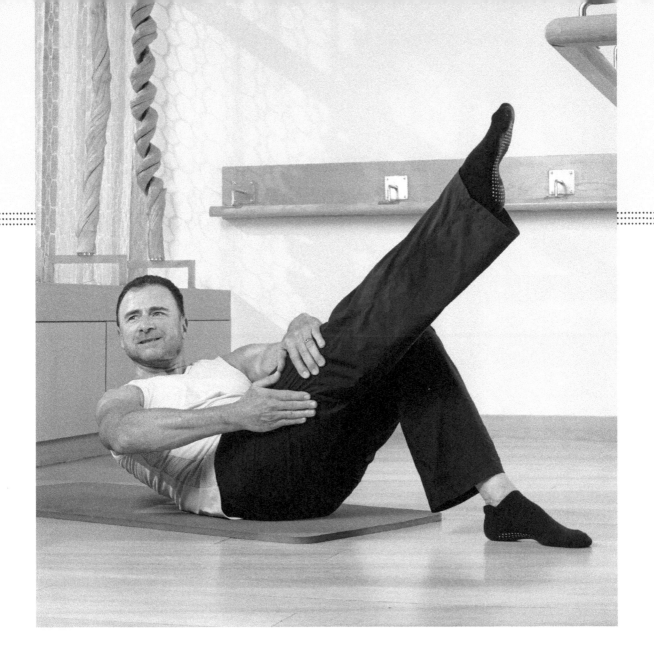

SINGLE LEG AT 45 DEGREES

1. Hold the Starting Position.
2. Keeping your knees level, extend your right leg at a 45-degree angle.
3. Bring your left hand to your right outer thigh as you twist your upper body to the right.
4. Hold on with both hands and stay in the position without falling back or coming up.
5. Hold the position for 10 seconds.
6. Rest and repeat on the other side.

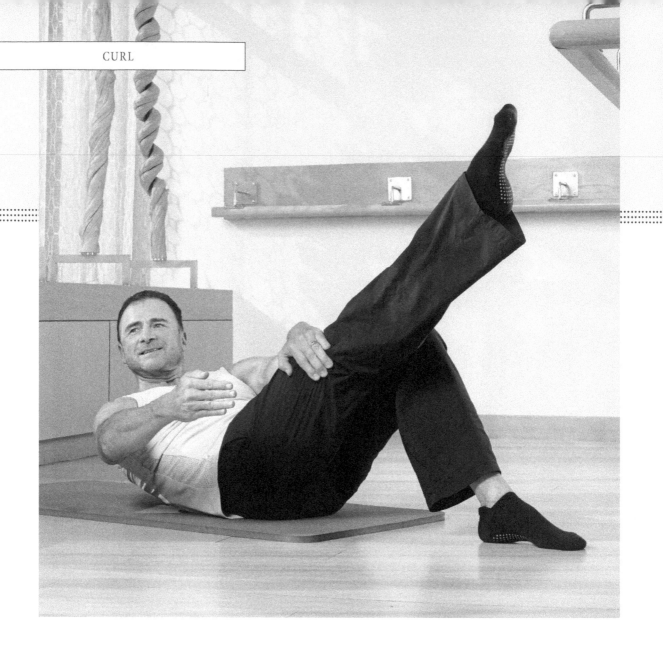

NEXT LEVEL (SINGLE LEG AT 45 DEGREES)

1. Establish the Single Leg at 45 Degrees position.
2. Take the bottom hand off your outer thigh without falling back or coming up.
3. Hold for 10 seconds.
4. Take both hands off your outer thigh without falling back or coming up.
5. Hold for 10 seconds.
6. Rest and repeat on other side.

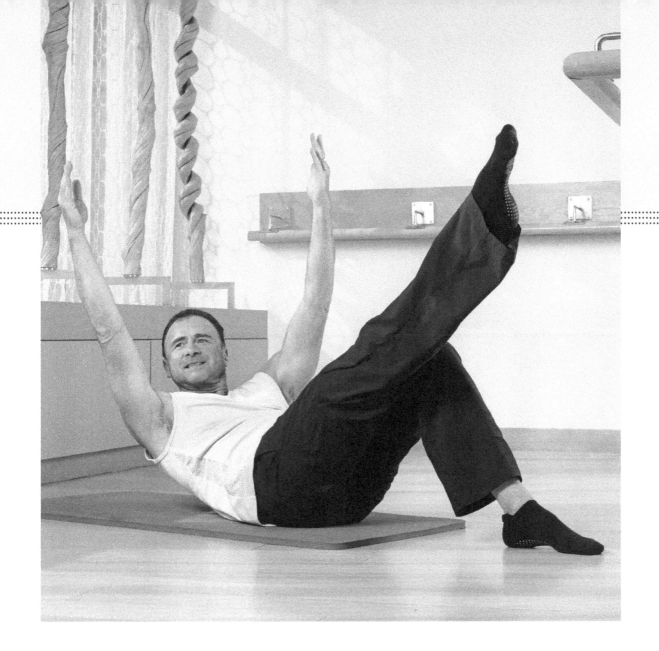

ADVANCED VARIATION (SINGLE LEG AT 45 DEGREES)

1. Establish the Single Leg at 45 Degrees position.
2. Take both hands off your outer thigh without falling back or coming up.
3. Hold for 10 seconds.
4. Raise your arms up toward your ears without falling back or coming up.
5. Hold for 10 seconds.
6. Rest and repeat on other side.

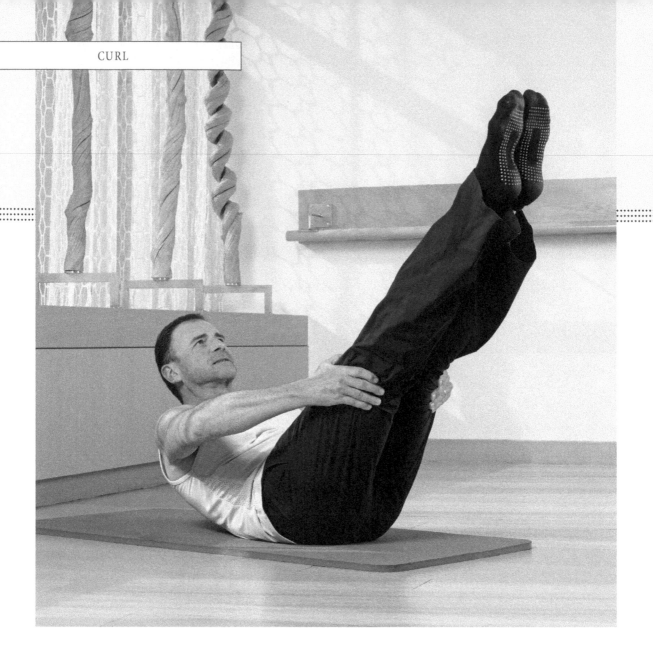

CURL

TWO LEGS AT 45 DEGREES

1. Establish the Starting Position.
2. Hold on with both hands and keep your elbows wide, your shoulders down, your chin open, your abdominals pulled in, and your pelvis tucked under.
3. Extend one leg to a 45-degree angle and then the other.
4. Hold on with both hands and keep your shoulder blades off the mat.
5. Hold the position for 10 seconds.
6. Rest and repeat 5 times.

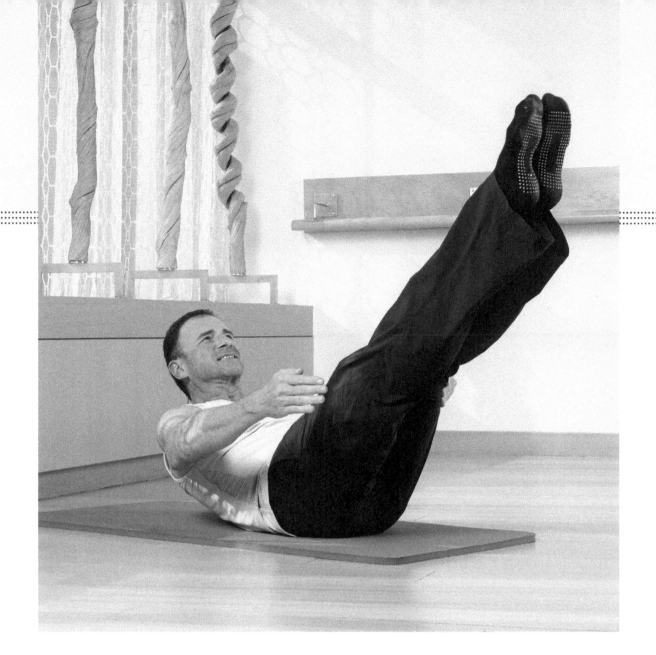

NEXT LEVEL (TWO LEGS AT 45 DEGREES)

1. Establish the Two Legs at 45 Degrees position.
2. Take one hand off your outer thigh and hold for 10 seconds without falling back or coming up.
3. Take both hands off your outer thigh and hold for 10 seconds without falling back or coming up.
4. Rest and repeat.

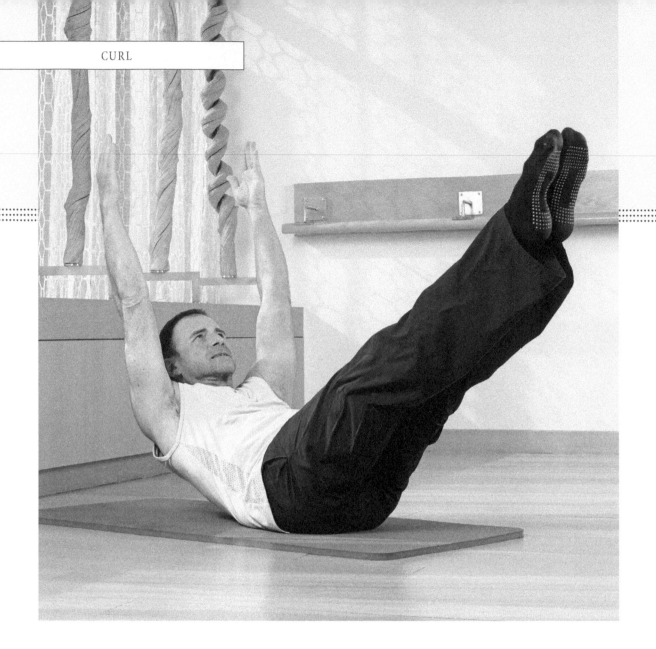

ADVANCED VARIATION 1 (TWO LEGS AT 45 DEGREES)

1. Establish the Two Legs at 45 Degrees position.
2. Take one hand off, then take the other hand off, and raise both arms toward your ears without falling back or coming up.
3. Hold for 10 seconds.
4. Rest and repeat.

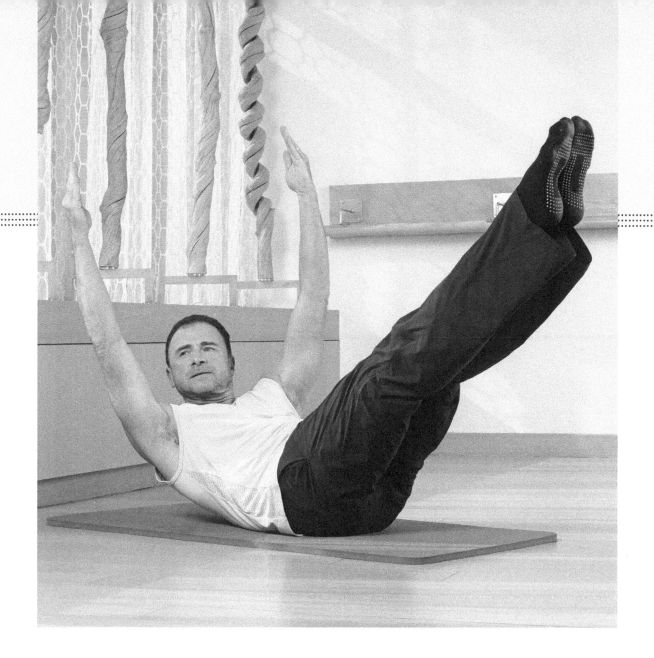

ADVANCED VARIATION 2
(TWO LEGS AT 45 DEGREES, OBLIQUES)

1. Establish the Two Legs at 45 Degrees position.
2. Take your right hand to your left outer thigh and twist your upper body to the left.
3. While maintaining the position and keeping your shoulder blades off the mat, take your bottom hand off, then your top hand off.
4. Raise both arms up without falling back or coming up.
5. Hold for 10 seconds.
6. Rest and repeat other side.

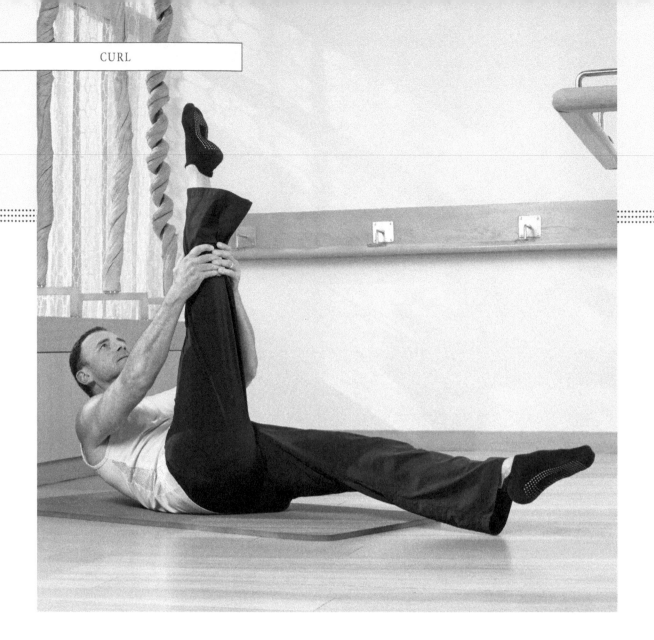

SINGLE LEG AT 90 DEGREES

1. Establish the Starting Position.

2. Hold on with both hands and keep your elbows wide, your shoulders down, your chin open, your abdominals pulled in, and your pelvis tucked under.

3. Extend one leg to a 90 degree angle and the other parallel to the floor and a few inches (7.5 to 10 cm) above it.

4. Hold on with both hands and keep your shoulder blades off the mat.

5. Hold the position for 10 seconds.

6. Rest and repeat 5 times.

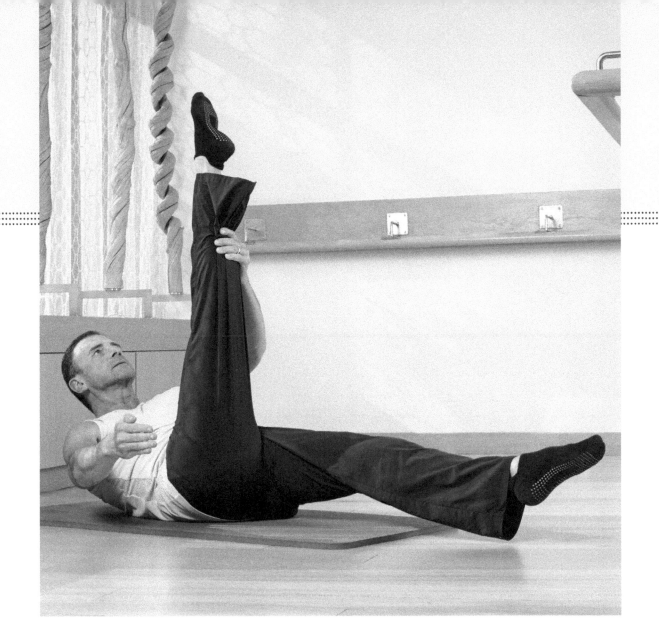

NEXT LEVEL (SINGLE LEG AT 90 DEGREES)

1. Establish the Single Leg at 90 Degrees position.
2. Take one hand off your outer thigh and hold for 10 seconds without falling back or coming up.
3. Hold for 10 seconds.
4. Take both hands off your outer thigh and hold for 10 seconds without falling back or coming up.
5. Hold for 10 seconds.
6. Rest and repeat.

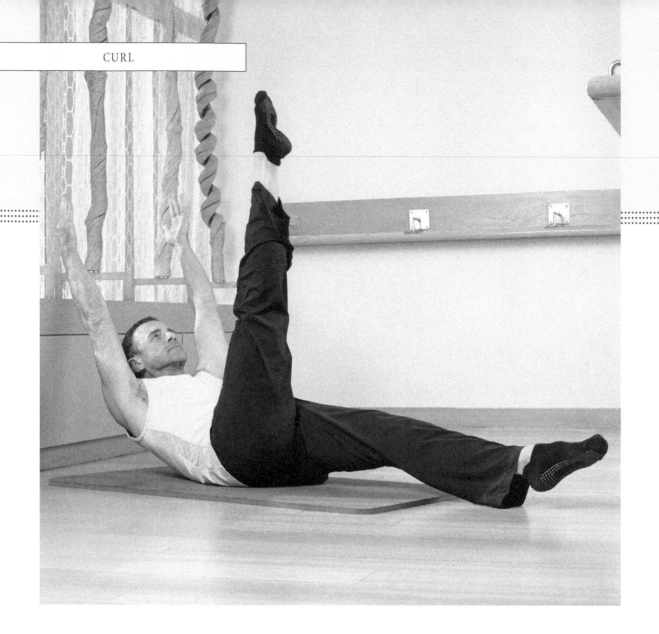

ADVANCED VARIATION 1 (SINGLE LEG AT 90 DEGREES)

1. Establish the Single Leg at 90 Degrees position.

2. Take one hand off, then take your other hand off, and raise both arms toward your ears without falling back or coming up.

3. Hold for 10 seconds.

4. Rest and repeat.

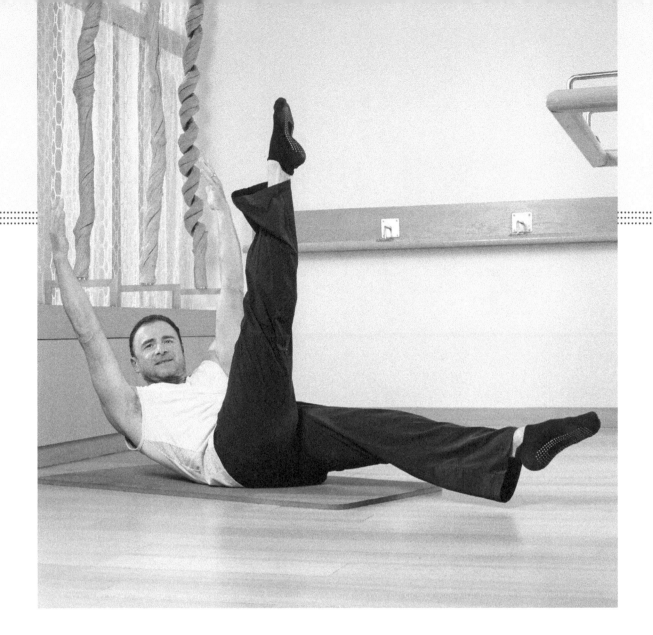

ADVANCED VARIATION 2
(SINGLE LEG AT 90 DEGREES, OBLIQUES)

1. Establish the Single Leg at 90 Degrees position.

2. Take your right hand to your left outer thigh and twist your upper body to the left.

3. While maintaining the position and keeping your shoulder blades off the mat, take your bottom hand off, then your top hand off.

4. Raise both arms without falling back or coming up.

5. Hold for 10 seconds.

6. Rest and repeat to the other side.

SPHINX

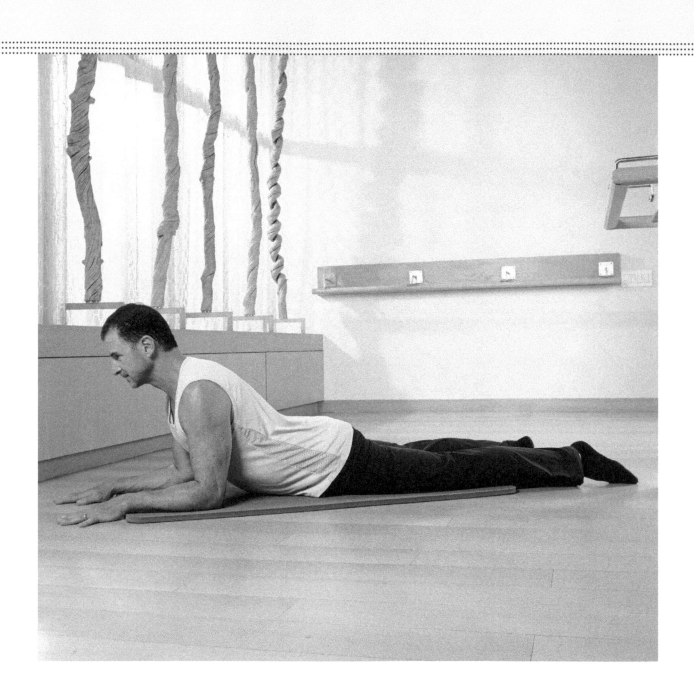

PRIMARY MUSCLES: The upper back strengthens as the abdominal muscles stretch.

STABILIZING MUSCLES: The shoulder girdle presses down.

This position will help you stretch the abdominal muscles and strengthen the upper back muscles. It will act as the counter pose to the curl. When dealing with spinal muscles, it is important to maintain a balance of strength and flexibility.

SET UP AND BASIC VARIATION

1. Lie on your front with your legs extended behind you hip-width apart.
2. Position your elbows under your shoulders and lift your chest.
3. Hold the position for 3 deep breaths.

WATCH OUT FOR
- *Elbows not in line with shoulders*

FIX IT
- *Realign as needed to be sure the elbows are directly under the shoulders.*

WATCH OUT FOR
- *Shoulders lifting up*

FIX IT
- *Reduce the intensity of the exercise and press your shoulders down.*

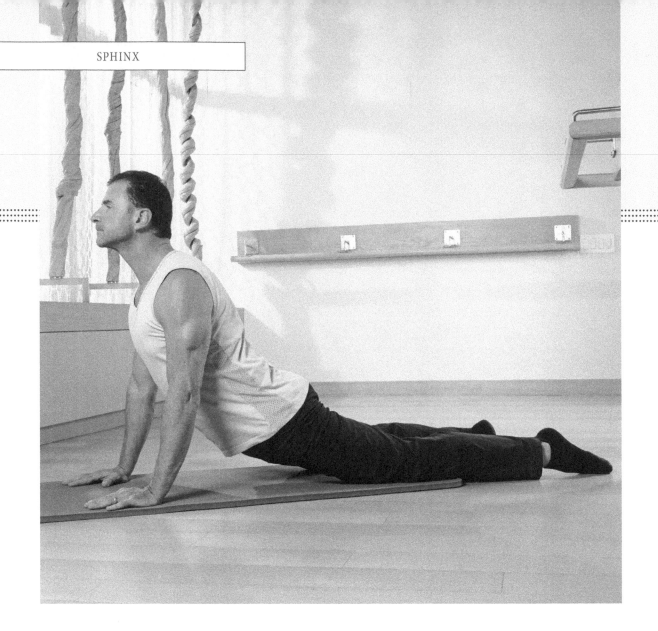

NEXT LEVEL (COBRA)

1. Assume the Sphinx Pose.

2. Lie on your front with your legs extended behind you hip-width apart.

3. Position your elbows under your shoulders and lift your chest.

4. Straighten both arms with hands under your shoulders, fingers pointing forward.

5. Hold the position for 3 deep breaths.

>Prone and Pelvic Tilt<
PRONE

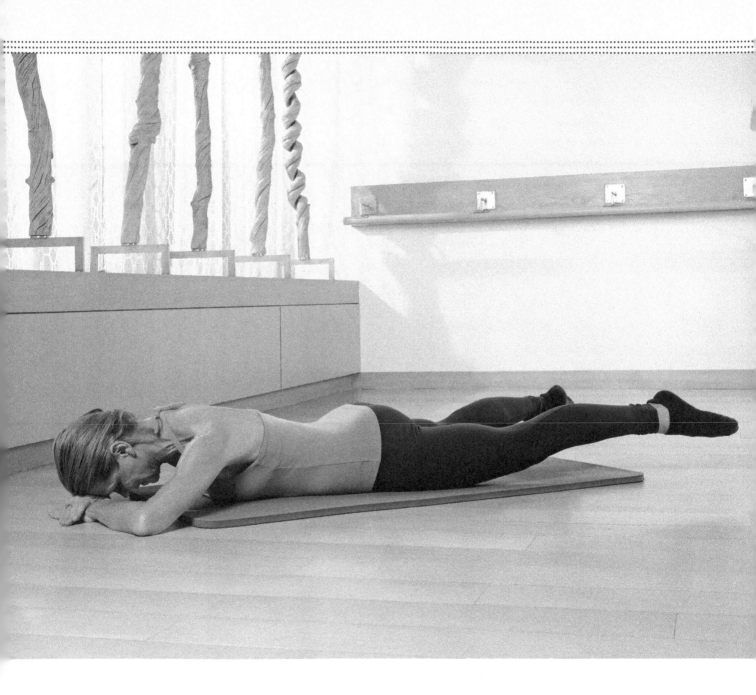

PRIMARY MUSCLES: The upper, middle, and lower back muscles strengthen.

STABILIZING MUSCLES: These are the same as the primary muscles above.

This position will help you build strength in your back muscles to form the perfect complement to the Curl, which stretches the back muscles. Keeping the back muscles strong will offer you more enduring postural support for your skeletal system.

SET UP AND BASIC VARIATION

1. Lie on your front with your forehead on your wrists and your legs extended hip-width apart.
2. Keeping your forehead on your wrists, lift your chest and upper body off the floor.
3. Simultaneously, lift both legs off the floor as well.
4. Hold for 5 seconds and release back to the floor.

WATCH OUT FOR
• *Overuse of the neck muscles*

FIX IT
• *Your head and neck should not move; only your arms and legs are lifted off the floor.*

WATCH OUT FOR
• *Lifting the head without lifting your arms and chest*

FIX IT
• *Your forehead stays on your wrists as you lift your arms and chest off the floor.*

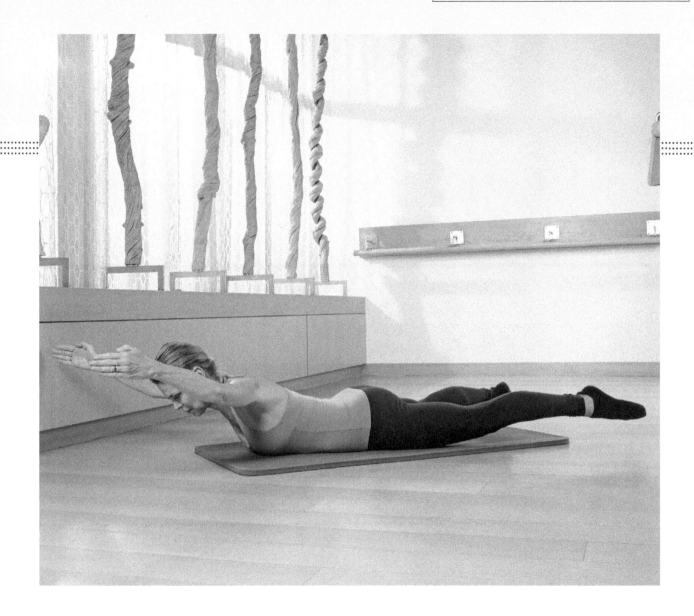

NEXT LEVEL

1. Assume the Prone Position.
2. Lift your chest and upper body off the floor with your arms extended in front of your shoulders.
3. Simultaneously, lift both legs off the floor as well.
4. Alternately flutter-kick your arms and your legs 10 times.

CHILD'S POSE

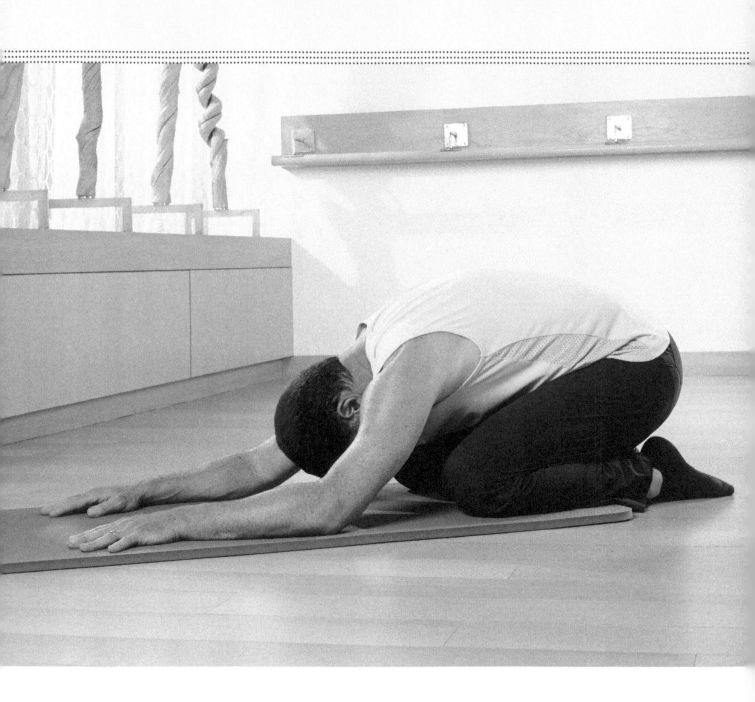

PRIMARY MUSCLES: The muscles of the back, especially the lower back, are stretched.

STABILIZING MUSCLES: The body is really not bracing here, so the muscles are relaxed.

This position is important to do right after the Prone back strengthener because it is a great stretch for the back, once more creating that counter-pose effect to balance your body.

SET UP AND BASIC VARIATION

1. From a face-down position, lift your hips and shift them back toward your heels.
2. Separate your knees wider than your hips as you sit back and extend your arms along the floor out in front of your shoulders.
3. Hold the position for 3 deep breaths.

WATCH OUT FOR
• *Knee discomfort*

FIX IT
• *Place a rolled-up towel behind the knees to reduce the bending in your knee joints.*

WATCH OUT FOR
• *Lack of flexibility making it a challenging position to achieve*

FIX IT
• *Open your knees wider and stay up higher as you bend forward.*

PELVIC TILT

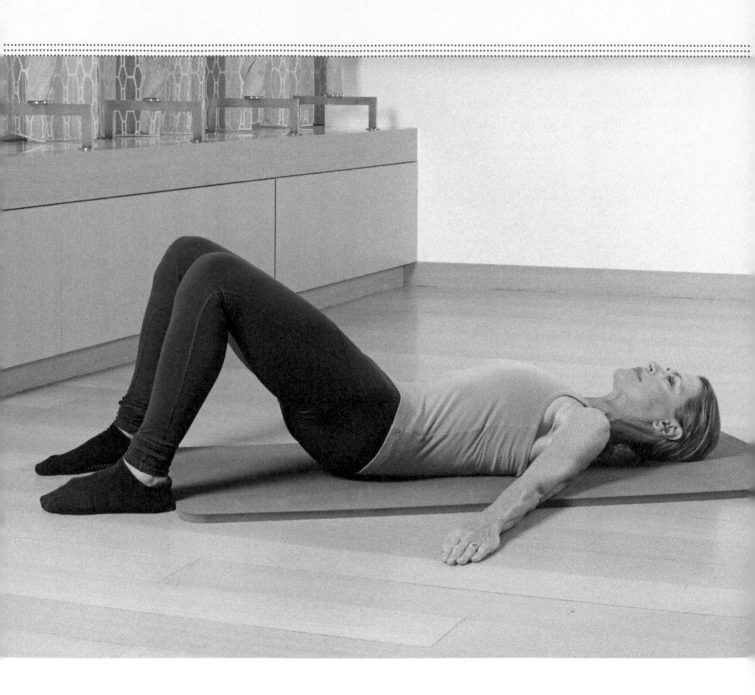

PRIMARY MUSCLES: The gluteals, hamstrings, inner thighs, and rectus abdominus are the primary muscles used in this exercise.

STABILIZING MUSCLES: The feet muscles, lower back, and abdominals are the stabilizing muscles used in this exercise.

The Pelvic Tilt helps to stretch the lower back and alleviate lower back discomfort. It also helps to strengthen the abdominal wall. This exercise is used a lot in physical therapy to help with lower back issues. It also helps to lift and strengthen the gluteals and hamstrings.

SET UP AND BASIC VARIATION

1. Lie flat on your back; bend your knees, making a 90-degree angle.

2. Your legs should be hip-width apart and parallel.

3. Place your feet flat on the floor facing forward.

4. Place your extended arms below your shoulders with your palms down about a foot (30.5 cm) outside your hips.

5. Keep your shoulders down and the back of your head resting on the mat.

6. Press your lower back into the mat.

7. Then do a very slight tilt up of your tailbone and engage your abdominals.

8. Release the tilt down.

9. Repeat the tilt up and down 30 times.

WATCH OUT FOR
- *Back arching or lifting lower back too high*

FIX IT
- *Press your lower back more into the mat and emphasize rolling your tailbone up.*

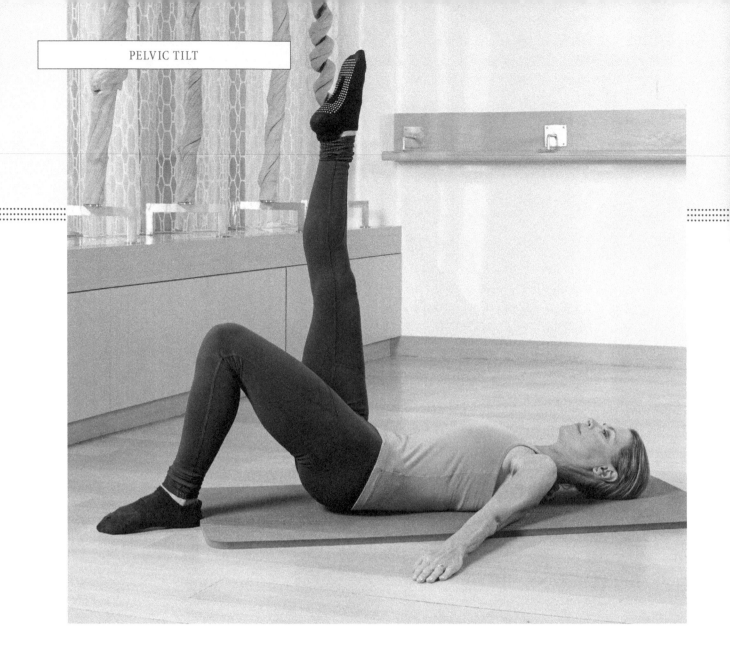

NEXT LEVEL

1. Perform the Set Up and Basic Variation.

2. Raise your straight right leg above your right hip.

3. Press your lower back into the mat.

4. Then do a very slight tilt up of your tailbone, keeping your leg straight. Engage your abdominals.

5. Release the tilt down.

6. Repeat the tilt up and down 30 times.

7. Repeat with your left leg extended above your hip.

PELVIC LIFT

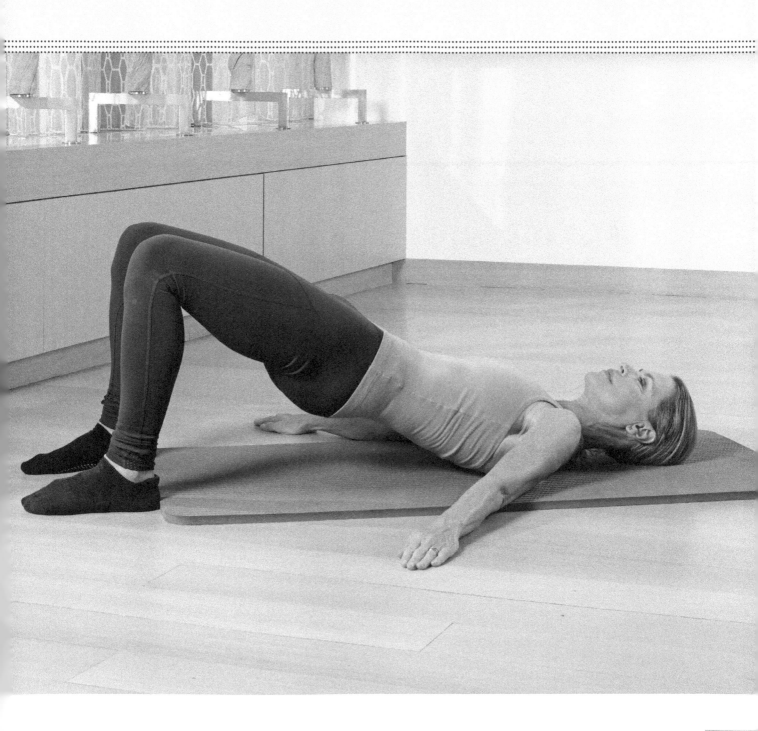

PRIMARY MUSCLES: The gluteals, hamstrings, inner thighs, and rectus abdominus are the primary muscles used in this exercise.

STABILIZING MUSCLES: The feet muscles, lower back, and abdominals are the stabilizing muscles used in this exercise.

The Pelvic Lift is similar to the Pelvic Tilt. It helps to stretch the lower back and alleviate lower back discomfort while it engages the length of the entire back, including the mid- and upper-back muscles. It also helps to strengthen the abdominal wall. This exercise helps to lift and strengthen the gluteals and hamstrings.

SET UP AND BASIC VARIATION

1. Lie flat on your back; bend your knees, making a 90-degree angle.
2. Your legs should be hip-width apart and parallel to each other.
3. Place your feet flat on the floor facing forward.
4. Place your extended arms below your shoulders with your palms down about a foot (30.5 cm) outside your hips.
5. Keep your shoulders down and level.
6. Rest the back of your head on the mat.
7. Press your lower back into the mat.
8. Shift your body weight back onto your shoulder blades.
9. Roll your shoulders down and keep them level.
10. Initiating from your tailbone, roll up one vertebra at a time to your shoulder blades/upper back area to complete the full range of spinal movement without an arch in your lower back. Keep your abdominals pulled in.
11. Then roll down with your upper back touching the mat first, then your mid back, and waist, and your lower back last to the mat.
12. Repeat rolling up and down 30 times.

WATCH OUT FOR
- *Back arching on the lift and lowering of back from the floor*

FIX IT
- *Emphasize rolling up, leading with your tailbone first, and leading down with the back of your waist touching the floor first.*

WATCH OUT FOR
- *Shoulders rising up*

FIX IT
- *Press the shoulders down and lengthen your arms down along your sides.*

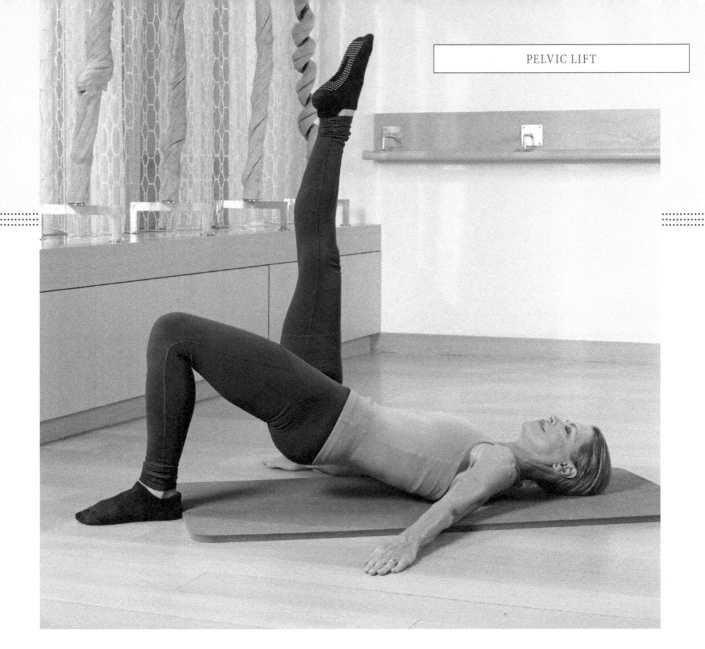

NEXT LEVEL

1. Perform the Set Up and Basic Variation.

2. Raise your straight right leg directly above your right hip.

3. Press your lower back into the floor.

4. Initiating from your tailbone, roll up one vertebra at a time to your shoulder blades/ upper back area to complete the full range of spinal movement without an arch in your lower back. Keep your abdominals pulled in.

5. Then roll down with your upper back touching the mat first, then your mid back, and waist, and your lower back last to the mat.

6. Repeat rolling up and down 30 times.

7. Repeat with your left leg extended above your hip.

> Final Stretch <

SAVASANA

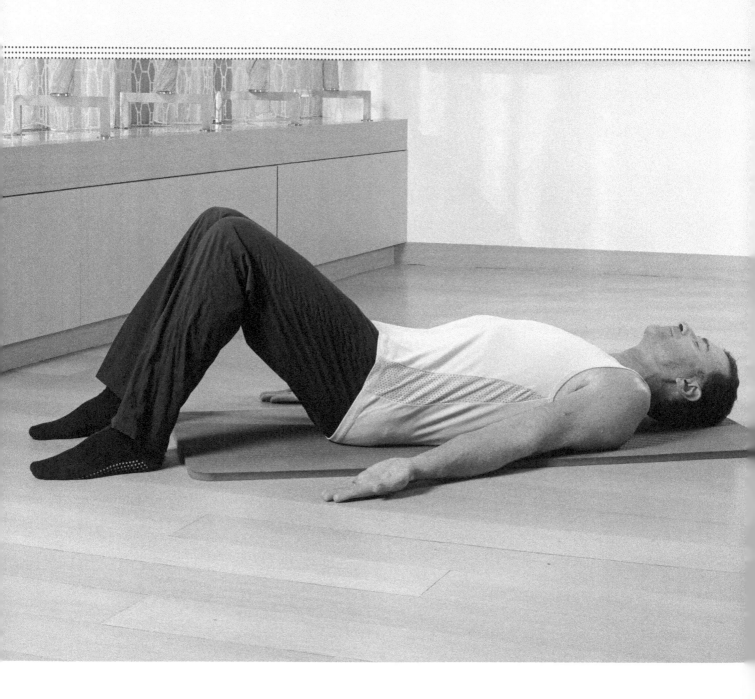

PRIMARY MUSCLES: None. Let all your muscles relax.

STABILIZING MUSCLES: None. Let all your muscles relax.

Savasana will totally relax all the muscles by lessening mental tension through stillness. Be sure to breathe mindfully and meditatively. This will allow the bones to sink away from the connective tissue. This relaxation of the entire body will relax the muscles. Focus on your breathing.

SET UP AND BASIC VARIATION

1. Lie flat on your back on a comfortable surface or mat.
2. Your legs should be bent at 90 degrees and hip-width apart and your feet flat on the floor.
3. Place your arms by your side wider than your shoulders with your palms turned up to be receptive to new energy.
4. Be aware of your breathing. Inhale 4 counts and exhale 4 counts.
5. Find stillness, surrender, and focus on your breath.
6. Stay in stillness for at least 3 minutes.

WATCH OUT FOR
- *Muscles tensing*

FIX IT
- *Exhale and let the muscles soften. Release your jaw, relax your face, drop your shoulders, relax your hands, soften your thighs, and relax your feet.*

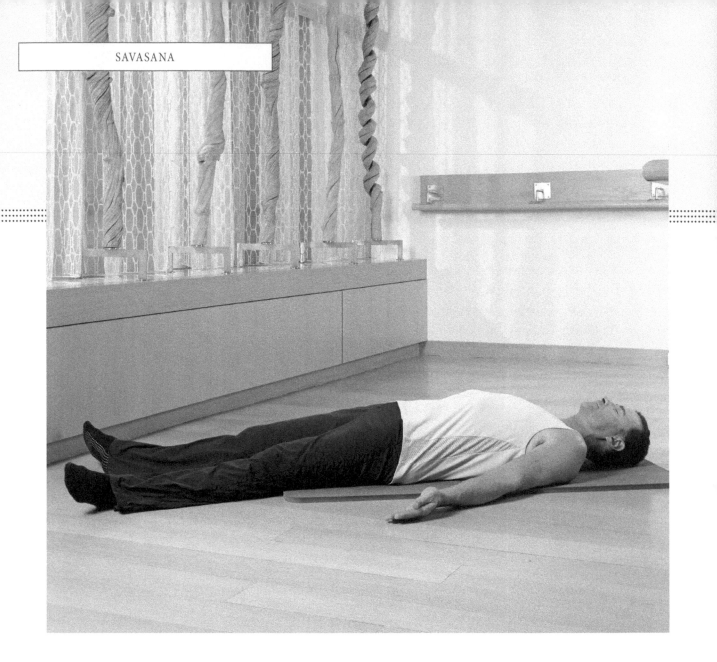

NEXT LEVEL

1. Perform the Set Up and Basic Variation.

2. Extend your legs straight and have your legs turn out naturally from your hips.

3. Stay in stillness for at least 3 minutes.

CROSSOVER STRETCH

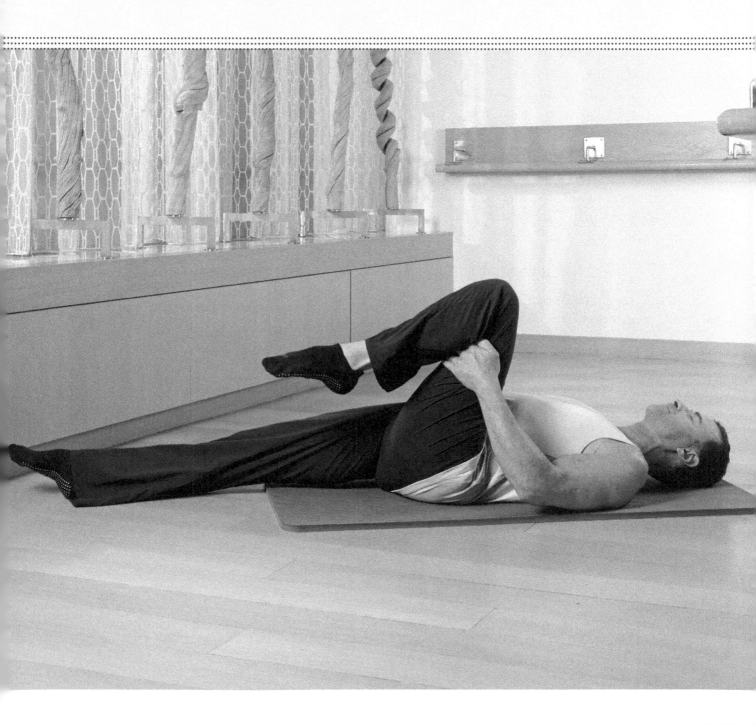

PRIMARY MUSCLES: This stretch lengthens the lower back and outer thighs and stretches the pectoral muscles.

STABILIZING MUSCLES: None, since you are on the floor.

This is wonderful stretch for the lower back, hips, and outer thighs. It helps to alleviate tightness from prolonged sitting and standing and activities that tighten the lower back. It is a great stretch for any sports that involve twisting, such as tennis and golf. We recommend doing this stretch every day. Remember to maintain a soft meditative breath and let the exhale take you deeper into the stretch.

SET UP AND BASIC VARIATION

1. Lie in a supine position with your back on the floor or a padded surface, with your ears, shoulders, and hips in alignment, and your legs hip-width apart.
2. Hug your left knee to your chest, holding on behind your knee on your hamstring with both hands.
3. Keep your right leg straight and extended.
4. Feel the stretch through your lower back and along the right side of your body.
5. Exhale and then continue to breathe easily.
6. Hold the stretch for 30 seconds.
7. Repeat with your other leg.

WATCH OUT FOR
- *Shoulders tensing and lifting toward ears*

FIX IT
- *Lower your arms.*

WATCH OUT FOR
- *Forcing the legs down to the floor*

FIX IT
- *Only lower your legs to where they fall naturally with gravity.*

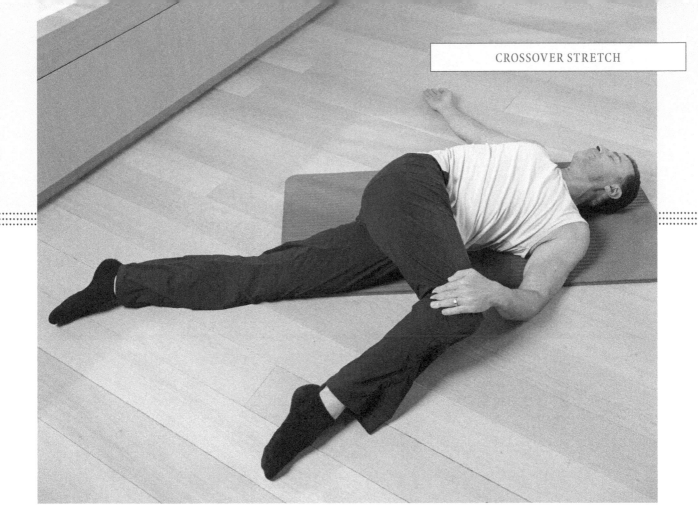

NEXT LEVEL

1. Perform the Set Up and Basic Variation.

2. Place your left hand on your right bent outer thigh and move your right leg to the left side of your body. Gently let this leg give in to gravity and lower it without strain.

3. Gently press your left hand on your right outer thigh.

4. Your right arm extends to your side down and below your shoulder. Keep your shoulders relaxed and down.

5. Look toward the right side of your body.

6. Exhale and then continue to breathe easily.

7. Hold the stretch for 30 seconds.

8. Use your left hand to bring your right leg back to your chest.

9. Repeat with your other leg.

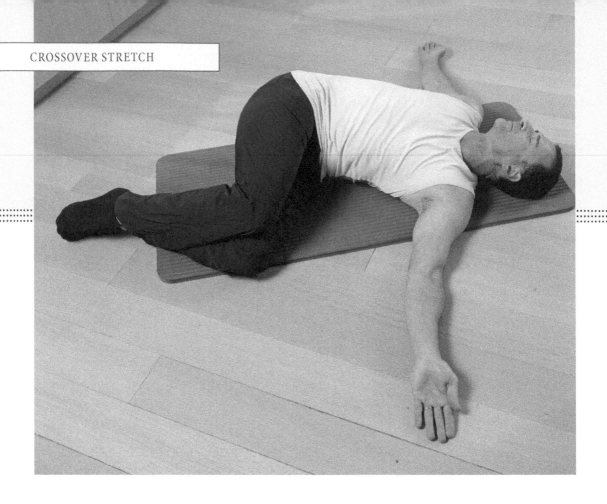

BENT LEG VARIATION

1. Perform the Set Up and Basic Variation.

2. Hug both legs into your chest with your hands behind your knees on your hamstrings.

3. Extend both arms to the side of your body below shoulder height, keeping your shoulders down.

4. Gently lower both bent legs to the left side of your body to where gravity takes them.

5. Keep your arms down; your right shoulder may lift a little off the floor. If you are able without straining your shoulders, try to keep both shoulders down on the floor.

6. Your head should turn toward your right side.

7. Exhale and continue to breathe easily.

8. Hold for 30 seconds.

9. Hug both legs back to your chest.

10. Repeat to your other side.

L-SHAPE LEG EXTENSION WITH BELT

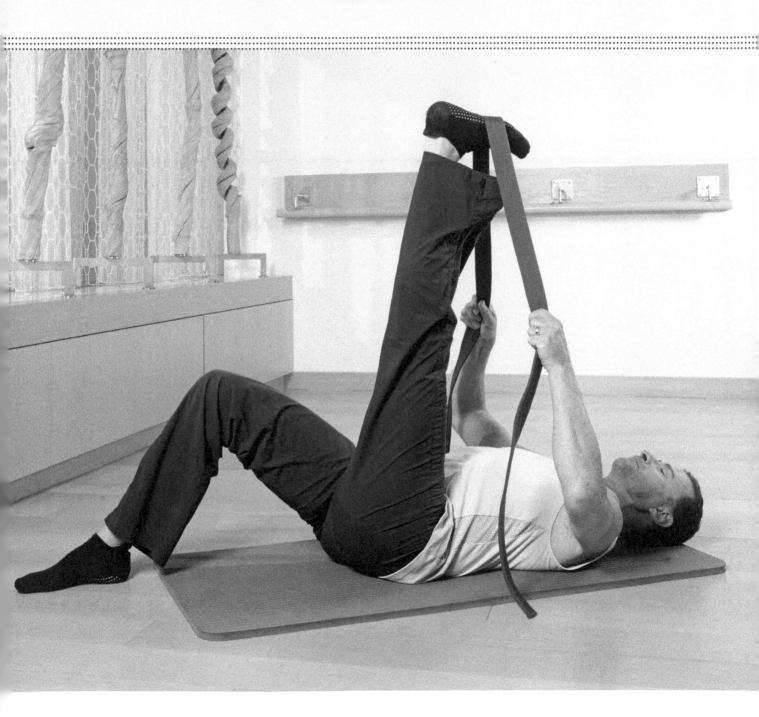

PRIMARY MUSCLES: This stretch lengthens the hamstrings, adductors, abductors, and calf muscles.

STABILIZING MUSCLES: None, because you are on the floor.

This stretch will use a stretch belt or towel to help get the full extension and length of the legs, creating a thorough stretch for your hamstrings, adductors, and abductors. This will help lengthen the muscles that get tight from sitting and any sport or activity that tightens the hamstrings, such as cycling and running.

SET UP AND BASIC VARIATION

1. Lie on the floor in a supine position.
2. Your ears, shoulders, and hips are aligned on top of each other.
3. Keep your knees bent hip-width apart and your feet flat on the floor.
4. Place the belt over the ball of your left foot and extend your leg above your hip.
5. Your right leg remains bent on the floor.
6. Place the ends of each side of the belt in each hand, allowing your shoulders to level out on the floor.
7. Engage your biceps instead of your shoulders to pull down on the belt, allowing your leg to press toward your chest.
8. Keep your lower back and gluteals on the floor.
9. Exhale and continue to breathe easily and mindfully.
10. Hold for 30 seconds.
11. Repeat with the other leg.

WATCH OUT FOR
- *Leg bending in the belt*

FIX IT
- *Lengthen the belt more to create more distance between your hands and legs to allow room for your leg to straighten.*

WATCH OUT FOR
- *Shoulders rising and tensing*

FIX IT
- *Press your shoulders down and level toward your waist.*

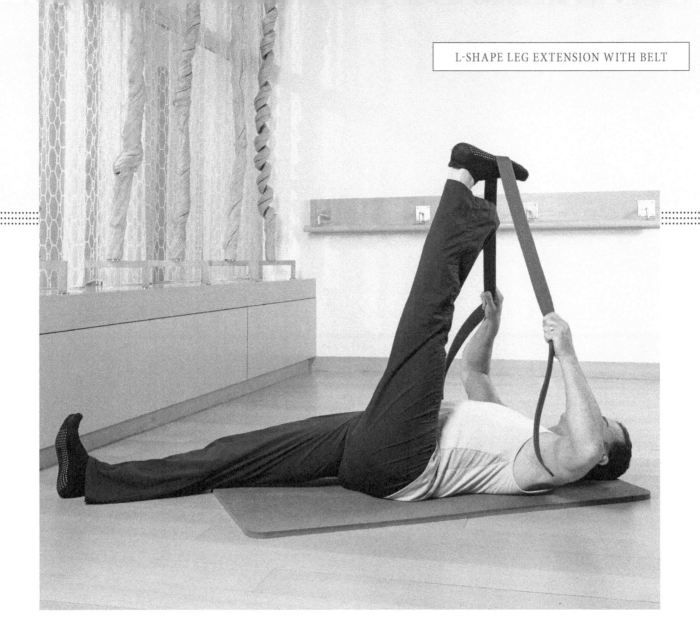

NEXT LEVEL, VARIATION 1

1. Perform the Set Up and Basic Variation.

2. Place the belt over the ball of your left foot and extend your leg above your hip.

3. Place the ends of each side of the belt in each hand, allowing your shoulders to level out on the floor.

4. Extend your right leg straight along the floor.

5. Exhale and continue to breathe easily and mindfully.

6. Hold for 30 seconds.

7. Repeat with the other leg.

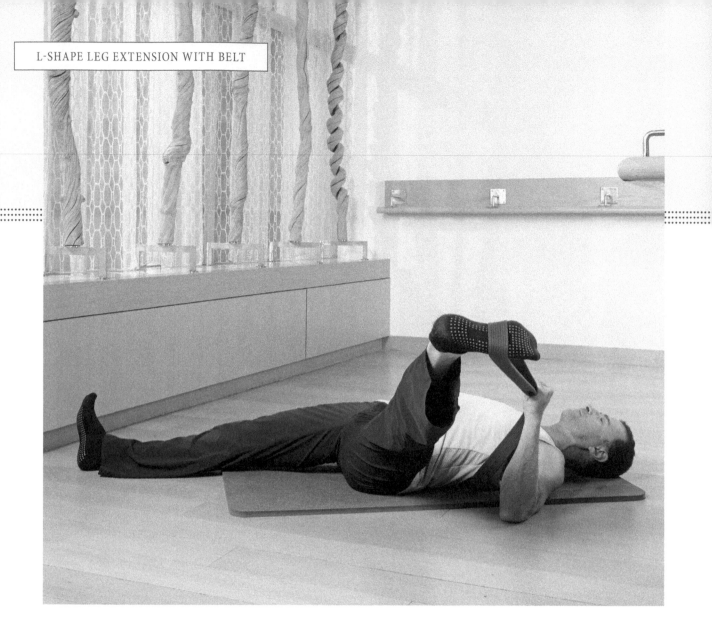

NEXT LEVEL, VARIATION 2 (OPEN TOP LEG TO SIDE)

1. Perform the Set Up and Basic Variation and Variation 1.

2. Place the belt over the ball of your left foot and extend your leg above your hip.

3. Extend your right leg straight along the floor.

4. Place the belt in your left hand.

5. Place your right hand on your right hip to keep your hips level and down.

6. Lower your straight left leg to the upper left corner toward your left shoulder for an adductor (inner thigh) stretch.

7. Exhale and continue to breathe easily and mindfully.

8. Hold for 30 seconds.

9. Repeat with your other leg.

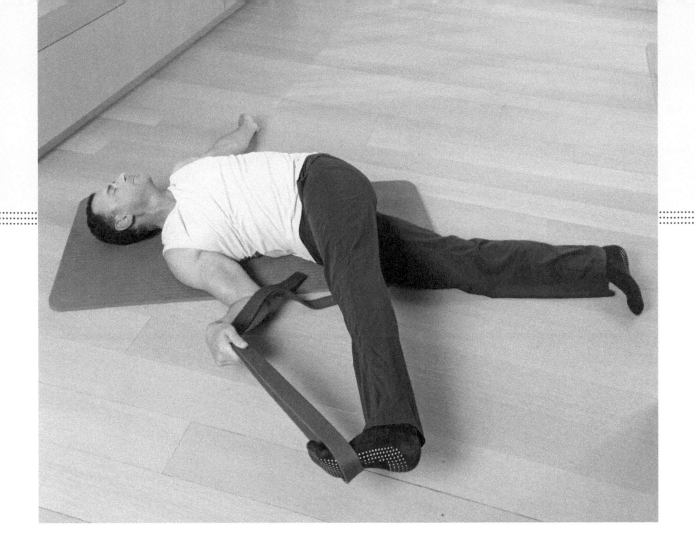

NEXT LEVEL, VARIATION 3 (TOP LEG CROSS OVER BODY)

1. Perform the Set Up and Basic Variation, Variation 1, and Variation 2.

2. Place the belt over the ball of your left foot and extend your leg above your hip.

3. Extend your right leg straight along the floor.

4. Place the belt in your right hand.

5. Your left arm should extend straight on the floor below your shoulder.

6. Move your straight left leg across your body, lowering your leg to your upper right shoulder for an abductor (outer thigh) stretch.

7. Have your left heel reach toward the floor with your toes facing upward.

8. Your left heel may or may not touch the floor; let the weight of gravity lower your leg to its maximum point.

9. Exhale and continue to breathe easily and mindfully.

10. Hold for 30 seconds.

11. Repeat with your other leg.

SEATED STRADDLE

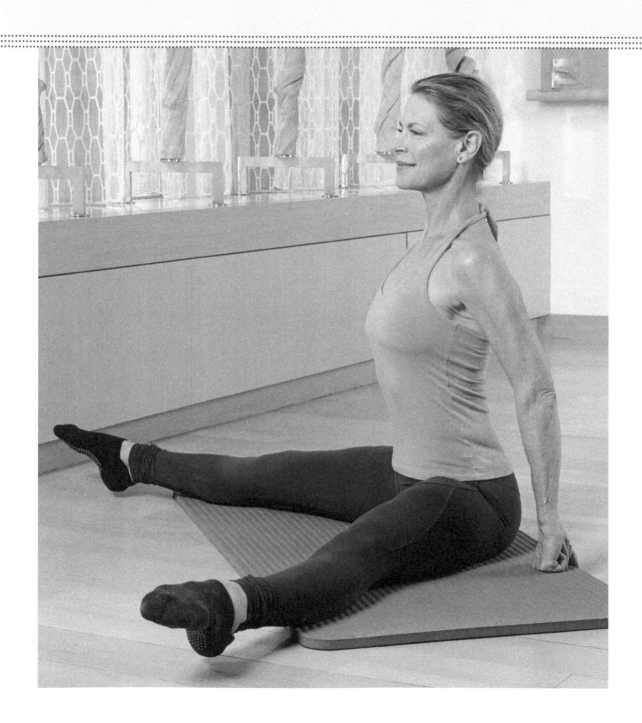

PRIMARY MUSCLES: The adductors (inner thighs), hamstrings, and lower back muscles are the primary muscles used in this exercise.

STABILIZING MUSCLES: The abdominals (front core) and side core muscles provide stability.

Seated straddle will help stretch the lower back, waist, inner thighs, and hamstrings. It will improve alignment and posture. Remember to relax and focus on your breathing.

SET UP AND BASIC VARIATION

1. Sit on the floor.
2. Extend your legs to a small V position with your knees facing upward.
3. Place your hands behind your body outside your hips with your fingertips touching the floor.
4. Keep your ears over your shoulders and your shoulders over your hips.
5. Your abdominals should be pulled up and in.
6. Point your feet.
7. Hinge forward from your hips, keeping your back very flat and straight.
8. Bring your hands or forearms to the floor. This will depend on your degree of flexibility in your hips, back, and inner thighs.
9. Gaze your eyes downward on a diagonal, keeping your neck in line with the rest of your spine.
10. Keep lengthening in your lower back on the exhale of your breath.
11. Hold for 30 seconds.
12. Roll up through your spine and hold your outer thighs to draw your legs together.

WATCH OUT FOR
- *Posture slumping forward from spine rounding forward and sitting into lower back*

FIX IT
- *Pull your posture back to a vertical spine by propping your hands on the floor behind your back plus bringing your legs closer together.*

WATCH OUT FOR
- *Side bend, opposite sitz bone lifts off the floor*

FIX IT
- *Reduce the degree of the side bend.*

WATCH OUT FOR
- *Side bend, shoulders rounding forward*

FIX IT
- *Keep your shoulders over your hips and bend less to the side and press your shoulder blades down and together.*

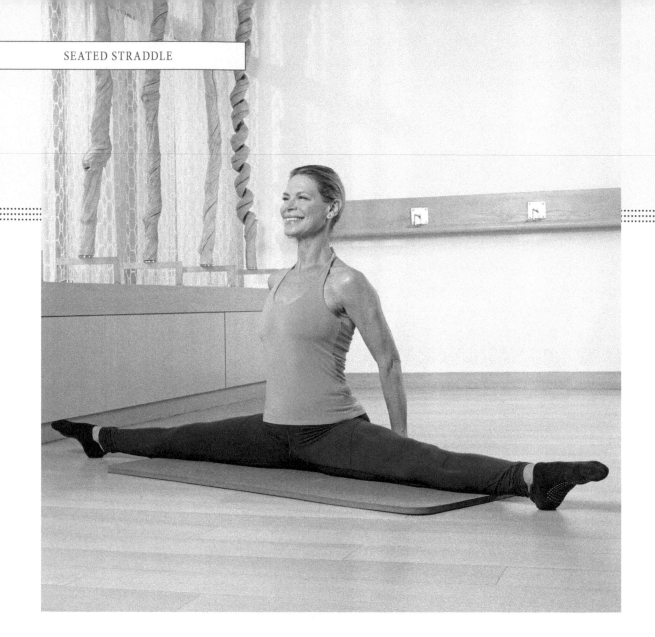

NEXT LEVEL

1. Perform the Set Up and Basic Variation.

2. Extend your legs to a wide straddle position with your knees facing upward.

3. Hold for 30 seconds.

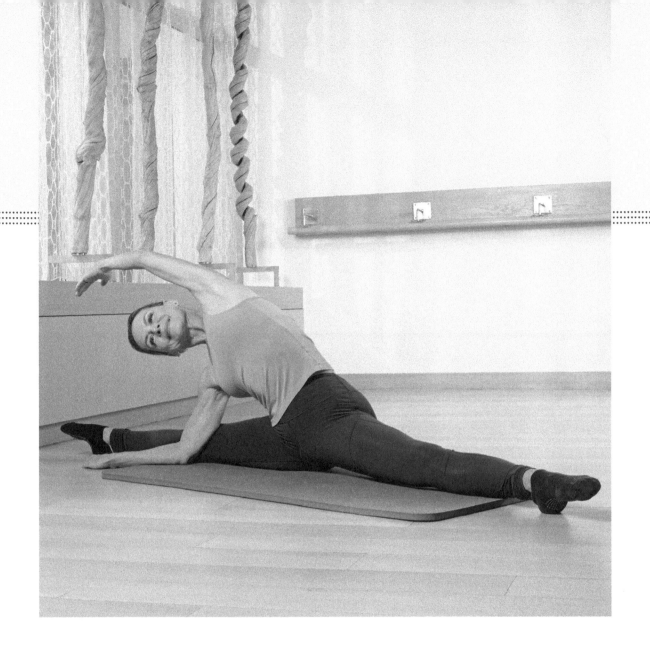

ADVANCED VARIATION 1 (SIDE BEND)

1. Perform the Set Up and Basic Variation.

2. Extend your legs wider if you have the flexibility.

3. From your Basic Variation or wider straddle position, raise your left arm and side-bend to the right. Keep your right hand behind your right leg.

4. Maintain the alignment with your chest open and your left shoulder back and down.

5. Hold for 30 seconds.

6. Come up and repeat to the other side.

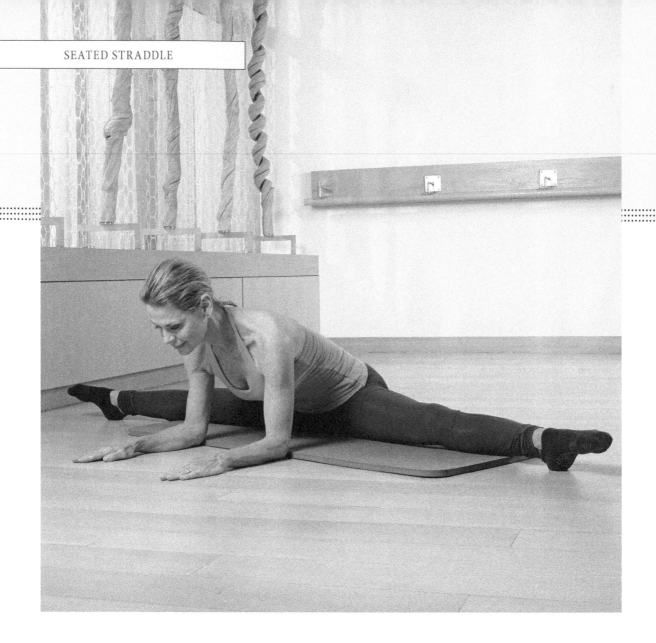

ADVANCED VARIATION 2 (FORWARD FOLD)

1. Perform the Set Up and Basic Variation.

2. Extend your legs wider if you have the flexibility.

3. From your Basic Variation or a wider straddle position, initiating from your hips and keeping a flat back, bring your hands or forearms to the floor or, if possible, extend all the way forward with your arms stretched out in front of you.

4. Only fold forward with a flat extended spine and avoid any rounding of your spine.

5. Hold for 30 seconds.

V-BALANCE

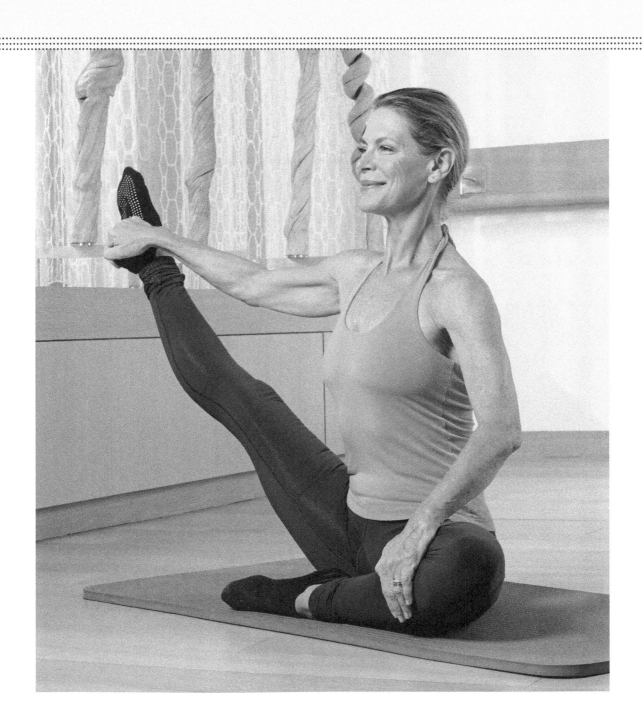

PRIMARY MUSCLES: The hamstrings, inner thighs, and back body muscles are stretched.

STABILIZING MUSCLES: The abdominals pull in and the shoulders press down.

This exercise is the epitome of stretch, strength, and core balance. This begins a pathway to balance. If the hamstrings are tight, your back may round over instead of forming a straight spine. At first, you may roll backward. Hold the calf muscle instead of the heel to reduce the height of the leg and enable you to obtain a more efficient posture. You need to first feel balance to find balance. By working on this position with patience, you will begin to understand how core bracing is the first step to achieving a balanced position.

SET UP AND BASIC VARIATION

1. Sit upright with your knees bent and your feet pointed in a V position. Place your right hand on your right heel or calf while your left hand stays on your left lower leg.
2. Extend your leg out to the side with the goal of straightening your knee.
3. Brace your abdominals in and press your shoulders down.
4. Hold the position for 3 deep breaths.
5. Repeat with the other leg.

WATCH OUT FOR
• *Rounding spine*

FIX IT
• *Hold your hand lower on your leg and keep your knee slightly bent in the beginning.*

WATCH OUT FOR
• *Shoulders lifting up*

FIX IT
• *Reduce the intensity of the exercise and press your shoulders down.*

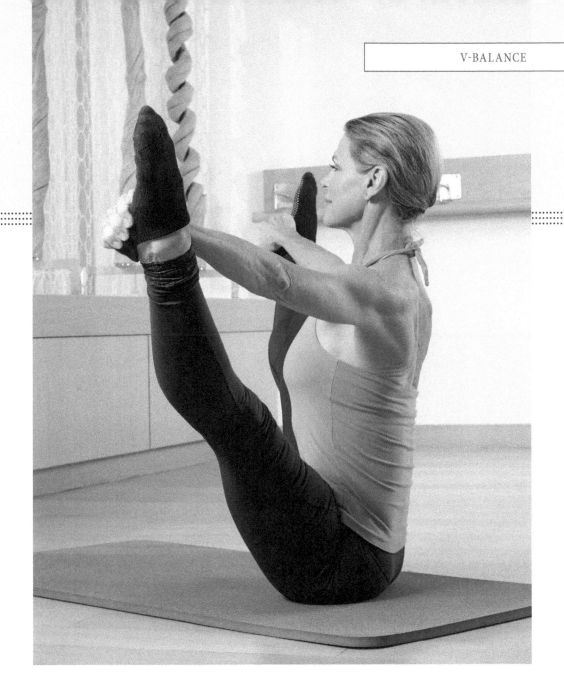

NEXT LEVEL (TWO LEGS OUT TO THE SIDE)

1. Perform the Set Up and Basic Variation.

2. Lean back slightly while bracing your core and take both feet off the floor.

3. Extend both legs out to the sides, trying to get both legs straight.

4. Straighten your spine as much as possible.

5. Hold for 3 deep breaths.

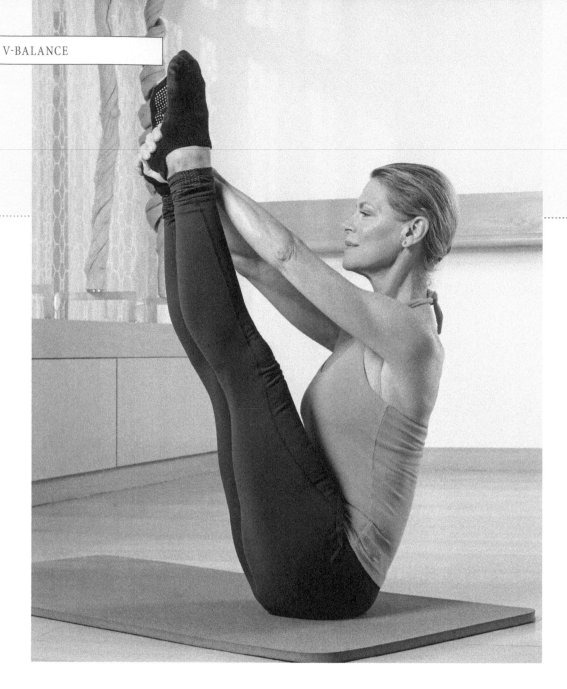

ADVANCED (TWO LEGS TOGETHER)

1. Perform the Next Level position.
2. Lean back slightly while bracing your core and hold your legs out to the side.
3. Slowly bring your legs toward the midline.
4. Attempt to straighten your legs and spine as much as possible.
5. Hold for 3 deep breaths.

GLOSSARY

CHILD'S POSE: Child's pose is a position in which you sit on your heels with your feet together, your knees open, and your upper body folded forward down the center.

EXTEND: When you open the angle of a joint, you are extending that joint. (Going from a bent knee to a straight leg is extending your knee.)

FLEX: When you close the angle of a joint, you are flexing that joint. (Bringing your toes toward your shin is flexing your foot.)

HIPS SQUARE: This is when both of your hips are facing in the same direction. Visualize the image of two headlights of a car pointing forward. This is an important consideration when exercising in proper position and alignment.

NEUTRAL SPINE: This occurs when the spine has its natural curves but particularly the natural curve of the lower back. When you tuck your pelvis under as one extreme and arch your lower back as the opposite extreme, a neutral spine is somewhere in between those two points.

PARALLEL: This is a stance where the feet look like the number 11. Usually, the feet are placed together or hip-width apart and parallel for a barre position.

PELVIC FLOOR: The pelvic floor consists of the deepest muscles of the pelvis located between the two sitz bones from side to side and between the bases of the sacrum posteriorly and the pubic bone anteriorly.

PELVIC TUCK: This is a position of the pelvis and is also known as a posterior pelvic tilt. A pelvic tuck is established by dropping the tailbone down and pulling the abdominals up and in toward your spine.

PLANK REFERENCE: When executing the plank exercise, try to remember what it feels like to hold your abdominal muscles in close to your spine. When you pull your abdominal muscles in, it should feel like a natural girdle around your waist. This feeling will be called for when you execute all of the other exercises that require core bracing and stabilizing. The feeling of the engaged abdominals pulling in is the correct way to stabilize and brace most exercise positions in this book.

PLIÉ: A plié is a movement in which a dancer bends the knees and straightens them again, usually with the hips turned out and the heels pressed together.

POINT: When you extend your toes away from your shin, you are pointing your foot.

POSTURE: In a standing position, proper posture is ears over shoulders over hips over heels. Exercising with proper posture provides lifestyle benefits such as less joint pain, more energy, better balance, and higher levels of efficiency.

PULL IN ABDOMINALS: This position is achieved when you bring your abdominal muscles in toward your spine. It is also known as abdominal bracing or abdominal stabilizing.

SHALLOW BREATHING: This is breathing high up in the lungs, in the thoracic cavity, and not allowing the abdominal area to expand when you inhale.

SITZ BONES: These are the small bones at the base of your body that anchor you to the floor or chair when you sit.

STANCE: This is how you place your feet on the floor to begin a standing barre position.

V- TURNOUT: This is a stance where your feet look like a narrow letter V. The heels are together and lifted a few inches (7.5 to 10 cm) off the floor and the toes are approximately 4 to 5 inches (10 to 13 cm) apart. The turnout happens from the hips.

WIDE SECOND: This is a stance where the feet are wider than hip-width apart in a V shape. The heels are either flat or lifted a few inches (7.5 to 10 cm) off the floor, and the turnout happens from the hips.

WORK ZONE VERSUS COMFORT ZONE: This is a concept that allows for the consideration of exercise intensity. Without intensity, there can be no results. It is important that the reader understand that when you are doing the exercises correctly, they will not be comfortable and will feel challenging.

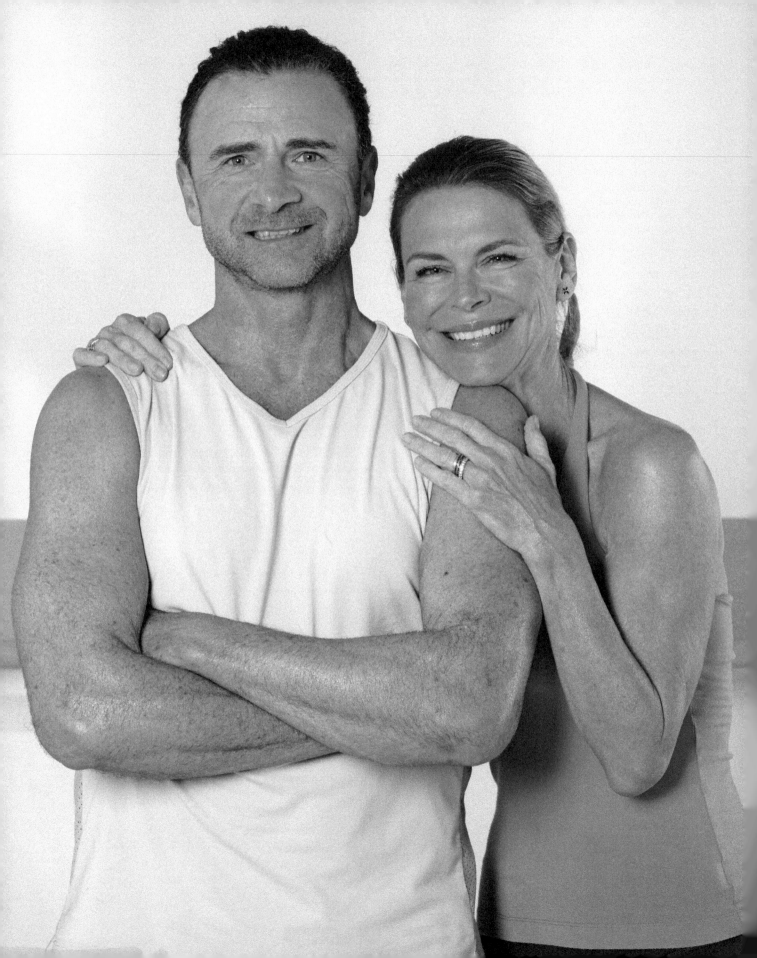

ABOUT THE AUTHORS

Fred DeVito grew up on the athletic field, where his love for sports led him to a life-long interest in movement science. He studied at The College of New Jersey, where he received a B.S. in physical education and health. Fred went on to become ACE–certified and teach physical education in the New Jersey public school system and fitness classes at local health clubs.

His wife, **Elisabeth Halfpapp**, received her degree in dance education from the Hartford Ballet. Later, she found a passion for yoga and became certified as a Yoga Alliance Teacher. Elisabeth's professional dance career kicked-off in the 1970s when she joined the Mercer Ballet, the Princeton Ballet (now the American Repertory Theater), Hartford Ballet, and Dances Patrelle.

Fred and Lis joined forces to become the faces of the Lotte Berk Method in NYC for more than 20 years. There, they built the acclaimed reputation of this unique and innovative Lotte Berk brand and technique.

After years of cultivating a local business and following, Fred and Elisabeth were eager to bring this life-changing fitness experience to a broader audience. In 2000, a Lotte Berk student, Annbeth Eschbach, approached them with a ground-breaking concept: merging authentic, result-producing fitness classes with holistic spa therapies and energetic healing programs. This concept already had a name: exhale. Fred and Elisabeth believed in Annbeth's vision and developed Core Fusion, an innovative, modernized technique with foundations based on the Lotte Berk Method. The first Exhale mind body spa opened its doors in New York in 2002 and has since debuted 27 locations (and growing) in the U.S. and the Turks and Caicos Islands.

The award-winning Core Fusion program and its suite of classes, including Core Fusion Barre, Core Fusion Yoga, Core Fusion Sport, Core Fusion Cardio, Core Fusion Boot Camp, and Core Fusion Extreme (H.I.I.T. class) are exhale's proprietary fitness classes, offered in most exhale locations in the U.S. and the Turks and Caicos Islands. Together, Fred and Elisabeth have created, choreographed, and starred in 11 Core Fusion DVDs and have contributed to many online classes on YogaVibes.com and other streaming video portals.

Based in New York City, Fred and Lis teach classes daily, lead well-being workshops and retreats nationwide, and continue to develop and train the signature exhale therapy, Thai Stretch, as well as direct exhale's Teacher Training Program, which trains dozens of teachers each year. In their newly launched 40-hour exhale barre teacher training program for community teachers, they train a few hundred teachers per year nationwide (in addition to training all of the proprietary Core Fusion teachers).

As lead trainers and fitness experts in the barre and well-being industry, Fred and Lis regularly appear as fitness experts on national TV including *The Today Show, ABC News, Fox News, CBS Morning Show, Entertainment Tonight,* and *Dr. Oz.* They have been featured in *The New York Times, Vogue, Fitness* magazine, *New York* magazine, *Glamour, Prevention, Hamptons* magazine, *USA Today, More* magazine, *Shape,* and *Women's Health* magazine. They share Core Fusion and yoga teachings with many charitable organizations regularly, including Mariska Hargitay's Joyful Heart Foundation and the American Red Heart Association.

For more information about exhale's barre teacher training program, visit www.exhalespa.com.

ACKNOWLEDGMENTS

We have a few important people in our lives whose guidance, encouragement, and love gave us this amazing opportunity to share health, well-being, and barre fitness with the world.

Together we would like to thank:

Lotte Berk—Although we never had the privilege of meeting Lotte, if it wasn't for her there would not be a barre fitness industry and the recent craze for these amazing exercises and positions. A lot of what Lotte taught back in the 1960s is still the backbone of what we teach today, simply because it works! Her small studio in London was the training ground of our first barre mentor, Lydia Bach.

Lydia Bach—Although she wasn't a fitness professional by trade, her ability to learn what Lotte shared and then bring it to the U.S.A. was unprecedented. It was her vision and directives that influenced how the upper echelons of NYC society women exercised and stayed in shape. For 20 years at her studio, the Lotte Berk Method, she was our most influential barre mentor and teacher. We learned how to teach a great barre class, run a business, train and negotiate with teachers, develop loyalty from our students, and be professionals in this industry. She taught us not only how to teach a great barre class, but also empowered us to share why these exercises were so effective.

Mino Argento—At the time, he was the husband of Lydia Bach and a father-like figure for both of us. Mino was the ultimate aristocratic, Roman–Italian gentleman who taught us the art of diplomacy. His sense of style and demeanor was the ultimate in cool, understated chic, and he nurtured our confidence to become great and respected leaders. He was the most skillful negotiator, often striking unbelievable business deals for the Lotte Berk Method that concluded with a winning situation for all parties involved. He was also a wonderful and brilliant painter as well as an eternal father and friend.

Fred L. DeVito—As a junior in high school and on the verge of making an important college decision, it was my dad who subtly recommended that I study to be a health and physical education teacher. He saw a vision that I couldn't see, but by trusting him and taking his advice, I followed a path that provided the backbone and skillset necessary for my work today as a teacher of movement and healthy lifestyle. He led by example, demonstrating with his balanced lifestyle how to be honorable, reliable, and consistent, which translated in my work as well as how I lead my life. Since his passing in 2012, I see his photo on the screensaver of my phone several times per day and call on his smile to soothe my soul and calm my spirit. His loving care while he was on Earth was my blessing, and his eternal love is my reality for which I will be forever grateful.

Nancy DeVito—I read tons of books on how to be peaceful, caring, giving, honorable, and compassionate. Books on how to let go of things that don't serve you, to focus on the good in people, and to send prayers of hope for those who do me wrong. But all of my readings shed a pale light on the one woman in my life who organically exuded all of these qualities and more. This is my mom, Nancy DeVito. Her wisdom, guidance, gentle advice, love, and care are demonstrated day in and day out by how she leads her life. Whenever I feel lost, confused, angry, or sad, it is my mom who brings me back to earth and grounds me. She rarely has anything profound or outrageous to say, just the simple messages and thoughts that bring good karma. She is my rock, and I am so blessed to have most of her genes for all of the loving qualities that make my life so full. I am grateful to have her influence in all that I do and all that I see in the world.

Elisabeth Halfpapp—My soul mate, my partner, my wife of 32 years, and my eternal love. As high school sweethearts, we began a life together sharing a love for so many things between exercise, sports, the outdoors, the arts, travel, and caring for others, that to say I am living a dream with Lis would be an understatement. She is the reason that I am in the barre industry and she loves to give me the "elbow in the ribs" when we team teach, often telling the students how she "hired and trained" me back in the day—which is totally true! As our careers unfold, we support and honor each other, sharing a sense of pride for all of the students and teachers that we have touched over the years. Our common bond is that we are in the business of changing lives. We feel so blessed to have an opportunity to give the gift of health and well-being to the world, and with any luck our mission and vision will continue to grow and flourish so that we can have a positive effect on those who cross our paths. She is my "core love!"

Christa Halfpapp—My mom was my best friend and passed away in 2000, too young at 60 years old. Because of her love of the ballet and opera, she enrolled me in my first ballet class at 5 years old, giving me the impetus to start my life in the ballet world that lead to the barre fitness world. She always gave me the freedom to choose any direction with my life, giving me support and love with those decisions. She nurtured in me my best alignment and posture, always telling me to stand up straight, shoulders back and down, and abdominals in! With her escaping from East Germany at the age of 16, she gave me the drive and strength that I could do anything I wanted with her famous words to always "smile and be nice;" every time I smile and stand at the barre, I think of her and her stately and humble manner. She loved to take my class and was always so proud of me. I miss her every day, but I feel her looking over my shoulder daily!

Bernhard (Ben) Halfpapp—My dad is still my best friend and always there for me, with love and care. We connect on the phone almost every night. His support has always been there for me, along with his incredible business mind and guidance. I truly believe that I inherited his uplifting people skills and smile; it is because of him that I feel my connection as a teacher to my students, along with having a hard time saying goodbye to people. I admire his incredible work ethic and he always tells me that you have to keep moving to live! He endured WWII in Germany as a young German child, and he inspires me every day with his incredible drive for life, survival, and physical strength. Dad, thank God you jumped out of the hospital window in Düsseldorf during the war before it was bombed or I would not have had such an admirable, loving, and supportive Dad!

Fred DeVito—My love, best friend, husband, and soul mate. I feel so blessed to share our lives together in giving health to so many people. Our hearts are one and we just move together organically as one. When I was 15 and his senior prom date, I just knew we were meant to be together the rest of our lives and that we would grow up together with heartfelt care, love, support, integrity, and in the fitness world. He truly is my other half and has enhanced and balanced my life in so many ways. I love him enduringly and deeply and hope to continue to move and dance together for eternity. With love to him from the core and barre!

INDEX

CPSIA information can be obtained
at www.ICGtesting.com
Printed in the USA
LVHW070954060220
646065LV00018B/596